KAMA SUTRA
WORKOUT

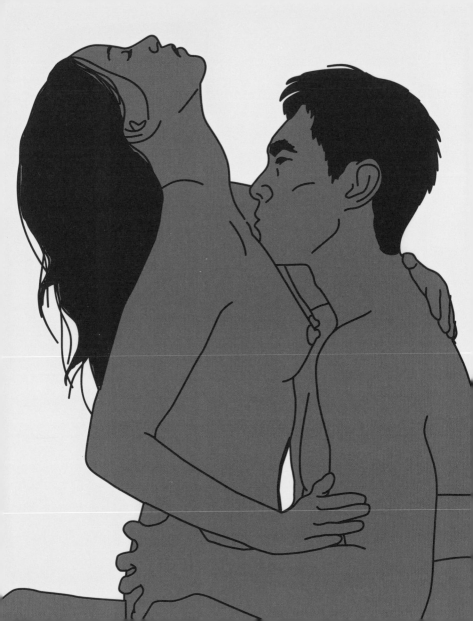

KAMA SUTRA
WORKOUT

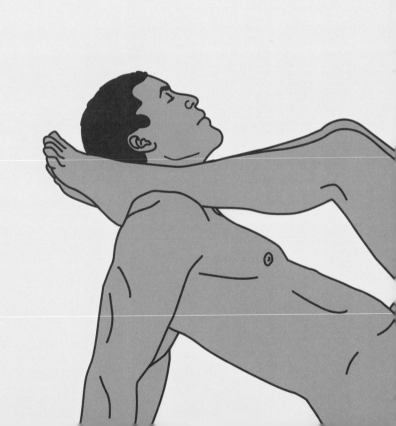

CONTENTS

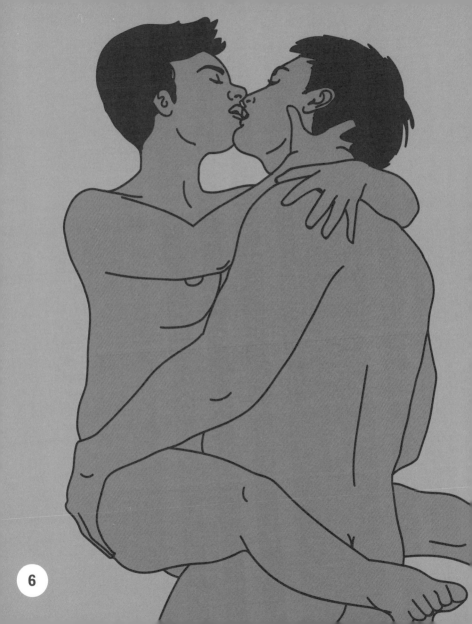

INTRODUCTION

You'll never want to skip your workout when it feels this good.

Inspired by the ancient wisdom of sex texts from *The Kama Sutra* and *The Perfumed Garden* to *The Ananga Ranga*, this book pairs **passion** with **fitness** so you can work and tone your body while reaching new heights of **sexual bliss**.

Each sexercise shows you which parts of your body you're working and includes stats for energy burn, flexibility, and duration. You can flip through and try whatever tickles your fancy; use the **position selectors** to find a sexercise that suits your mood; or, if you're both up for a hot and steamy workout, follow the **sex session sequences**.

In your pursuit of passion, don't forget that if it hurts, stop, and if you take your lovemaking out of the bedroom and into novel places, don't get caught.

There are 300 sexercises to choose from, so grab your partner, pick a position, and get a **sexy sweat on**.

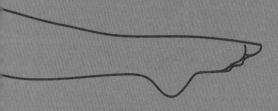

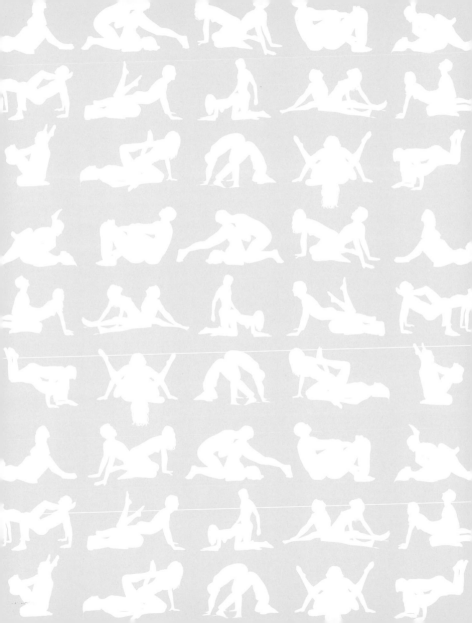

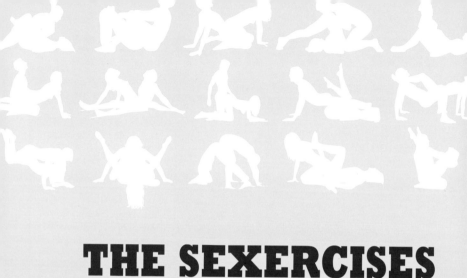

THE SEXERCISES

Discover something new, take inspiration, have a giggle: each of these sexercises will raise your heart rate and spice up your sex life.

KEPT IN SUSPENSE

You can both enjoy the erotic anonymity of this rear-entry position. One partner opens wide and you both go wild.

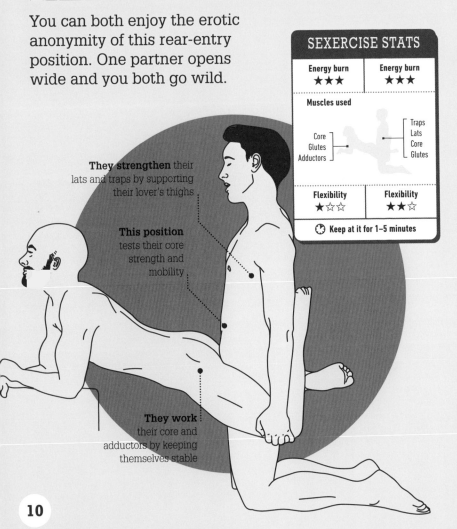

They strengthen their lats and traps by supporting their lover's thighs

This position tests their core strength and mobility

They work their core and adductors by keeping themselves stable

SEXERCISE STATS

Energy burn	Energy burn
★★★	★★★

Muscles used

Core
Glutes
Adductors

Traps
Lats
Core
Glutes

Flexibility	Flexibility
★☆☆	★★☆

🕑 **Keep at it for 1–5 minutes**

SIDE-SPLITTING SATISFACTION

Straddle your lover's thigh and enjoy an unusual angle. They can lift up their leg to let you in deep.

SEXERCISE STATS

Energy burn	Energy burn
★☆☆	★★☆

Muscles used

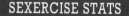

Glutes
Adductors

Core
Glutes
Hip flexors

Flexibility	Flexibility
★★☆	★☆☆

🕐 **Keep at it for 1–5 minutes**

You strengthen your glutes by thrusting forward

Maintaining this position strengthens their glutes and stretches their adductors

Your hip flexors stretch as you push forward

ARCH OF AROUSAL

This graceful pose requires strength and trust from both of you. Your partner loves feeling held firmly, while you admire their tantalizingly exposed body.

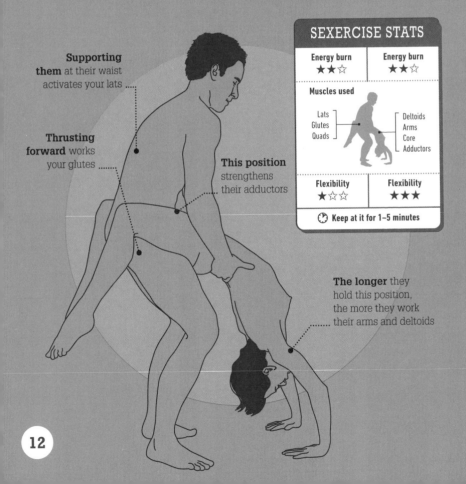

Supporting them at their waist activates your lats

Thrusting forward works your glutes

This position strengthens their adductors

The longer they hold this position, the more they work their arms and deltoids

SEXERCISE STATS

Energy burn	Energy burn
★★☆	★★☆

Muscles used

Lats
Glutes
Quads

Deltoids
Arms
Core
Adductors

Flexibility	Flexibility
★☆☆	★★★

🕐 **Keep at it for 1–5 minutes**

TUCKED UP

Create a tight and compact love knot. Show your lover where you want them, then pull them in close with your feet.

Thrusting forward
works their glutes

They get a
deep stretch
in their quads

You squeeze your
abdominals in this
compressed position

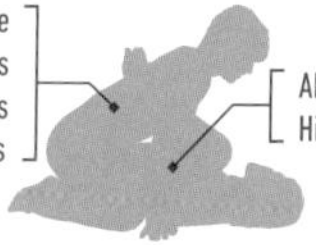

13

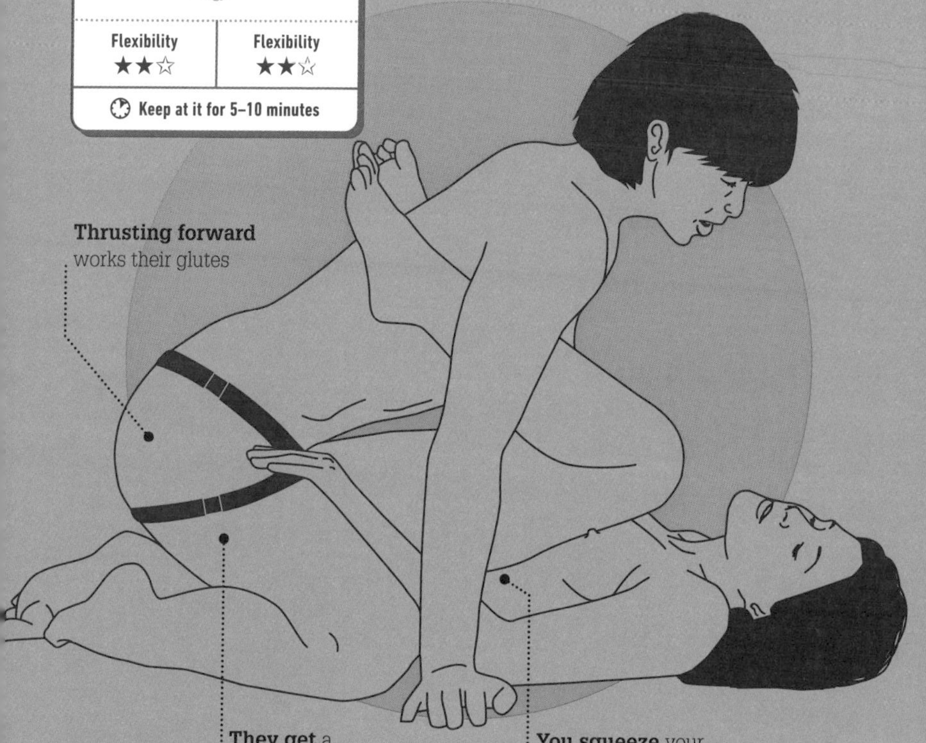

BEAUTIFUL BEHIND

Hold your lover's knees and rock yourself back and forth. The sight of your voluptuous buttocks gets them fired up and ready to explode.

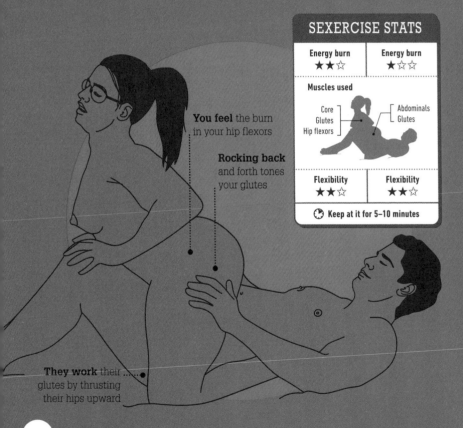

You feel the burn in your hip flexors

Rocking back and forth tones your glutes

They work their glutes by thrusting their hips upward

SEXERCISE STATS

Energy burn	Energy burn
★★☆	★☆☆

Muscles used

Core
Glutes
Hip flexors

Abdominals
Glutes

Flexibility	Flexibility
★★☆	★★☆

🕐 Keep at it for 5–10 minutes

X MARKS THE SPOT

Only the most crucial parts of your bodies touch in this explosive position. Once you are inside, they cross their legs to grip you tightly.

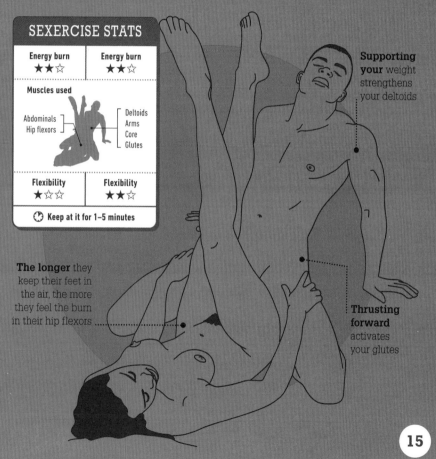

SEXERCISE STATS

Energy burn	Energy burn
★★☆	★★☆

Muscles used

Abdominals
Hip flexors

Deltoids
Arms
Core
Glutes

Flexibility	Flexibility
★☆☆	★★☆

🕐 **Keep at it for 1–5 minutes**

Supporting your weight strengthens your deltoids

The longer they keep their feet in the air, the more they feel the burn in their hip flexors

Thrusting forward activates your glutes

SEXPLORE

A naughtily novel position for ambitious couples.
Put your teamwork skills to the test and see
if you can rise to the challenge.

You activate
your abdominals
by holding a
forward fold

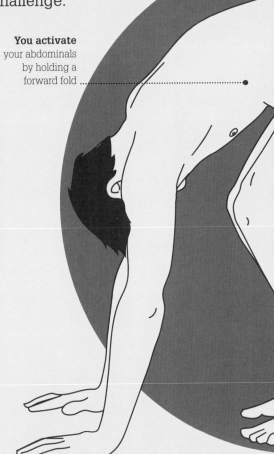

SEXERCISE STATS

Energy burn ★★☆	Energy burn ★★☆
Muscles used	

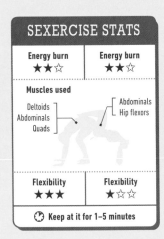

Deltoids
Abdominals
Quads

Abdominals
Hip flexors

Flexibility ★★★	Flexibility ★☆☆
⏱ Keep at it for 1–5 minutes	

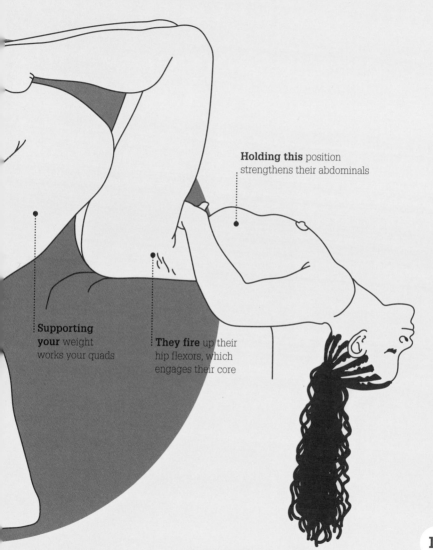

Holding this position strengthens their abdominals

Supporting your weight works your quads

They fire up their hip flexors, which engages their core

TAKE A SEAT

They give you all the attention in this intimate kneeling position—kissing your neck and using their hands will make you moan.

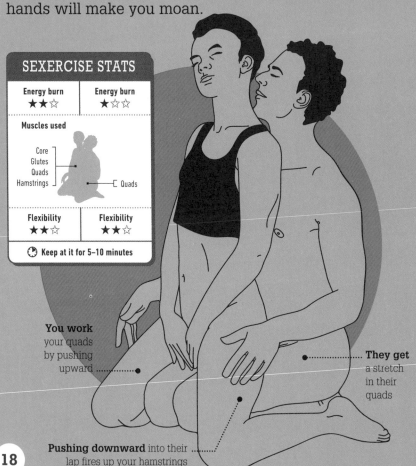

SEXERCISE STATS

Energy burn	Energy burn
★★☆	★☆☆

Muscles used

Core
Glutes
Quads
Hamstrings

⌐ Quads

Flexibility	Flexibility
★★☆	★★☆

🕑 Keep at it for 5–10 minutes

You work your quads by pushing upward ·············●

They get a stretch in their quads

Pushing downward into their lap fires up your hamstrings

18

LEGSTATIC

Your lover dangles their legs over your chest and frames your face with their feet. You grab their thighs and take it slow.

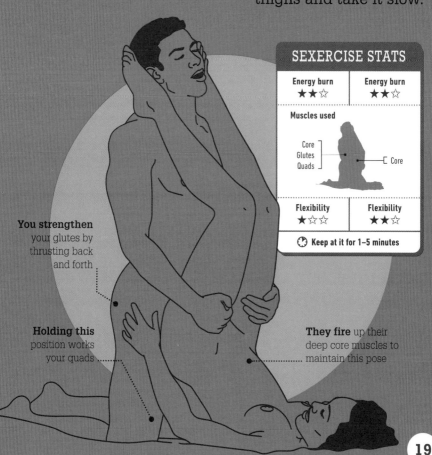

You strengthen your glutes by thrusting back and forth

Holding this position works your quads

They fire up their deep core muscles to maintain this pose

SEXERCISE STATS

Energy burn	Energy burn
★★☆	★★☆

Muscles used

Core
Glutes
Quads

Core

Flexibility	Flexibility
★☆☆	★★☆

🕐 **Keep at it for 1–5 minutes**

CUDDLE UP

For powerful but intimate sex, hug your partner from behind and wrap them in your arms. Hold their thighs and lift them up to take it to the next level.

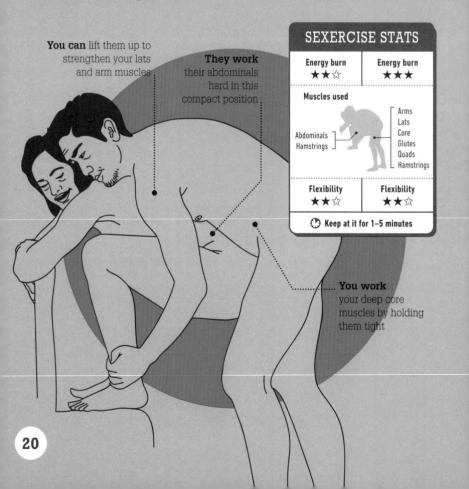

You can lift them up to strengthen your lats and arm muscles

They work their abdominals hard in this compact position

You work your deep core muscles by holding them tight

SEXERCISE STATS

Energy burn	Energy burn
★★☆	★★★

Muscles used

Abdominals
Hamstrings

Arms
Lats
Core
Glutes
Quads
Hamstrings

Flexibility	Flexibility
★★☆	★★☆

🕐 Keep at it for 1–5 minutes

A BIT ON THE SIDE

Hook your leg over your partner's thigh and lure them in at a side-on angle. Make it slow and sensual, or bump and grind against each other until you climax.

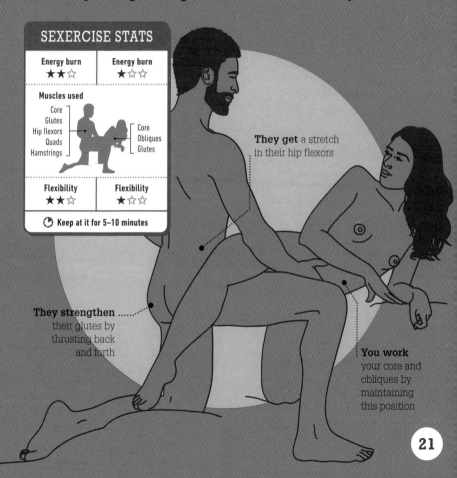

SEXERCISE STATS

Energy burn ★★☆	Energy burn ★☆☆

Muscles used

Core
Glutes
Hip flexors
Quads
Hamstrings

Core
Obliques
Glutes

Flexibility ★★☆	Flexibility ★☆☆

🕐 **Keep at it for 5–10 minutes**

They get a stretch in their hip flexors

They strengthen their glutes by thrusting back and forth

You work your core and obliques by maintaining this position

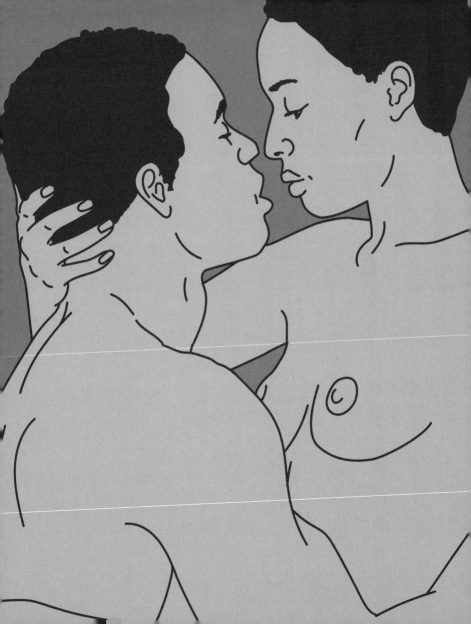

"ONE SHOULD *kiss* THE OTHER'S LOWER LIP AND THEN, BEING INTOXICATED *with love,* THEY SHOULD SHUT THEIR EYES"

THE KAMA SUTRA

PERFECT POISE

You take the lead by lunging over your partner, leaving them at your mercy. Stare into each other's eyes, but don't break the tension by kissing.

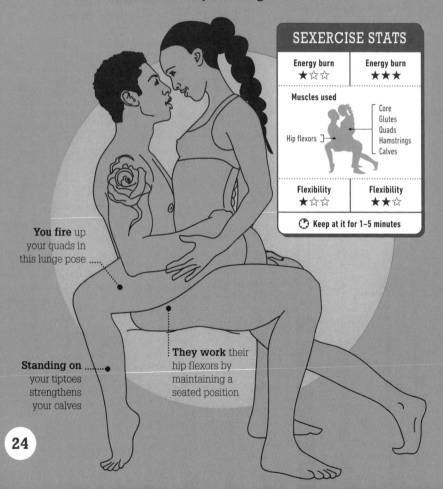

SEXERCISE STATS

Energy burn	Energy burn
★☆☆	★★★

Muscles used

Hip flexors ┤

┌ Core
  Glutes
  Quads
  Hamstrings
└ Calves

Flexibility	Flexibility
★☆☆	★★☆

🕑 **Keep at it for 1–5 minutes**

You fire up your quads in this lunge pose

Standing on your tiptoes strengthens your calves

They work their hip flexors by maintaining a seated position

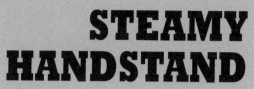

STEAMY HANDSTAND

Shake up your foreplay with a hot handstand. You trap your partner between your thighs until you're satisfied.

You contract your hamstrings and quads as you stabilize your body

You fire up your core and chest by supporting your weight

The longer they hold this position, the more their quads feel the burn

SEXERCISE STATS

Energy burn ★★☆	Energy burn ★★★

Muscles used

Biceps
Chest
Core
Quads

Traps
Deltoids
Chest
Core
Quads
Hamstrings

Flexibility ★★☆	Flexibility ★★★

🕐 Keep at it for 1–5 minutes

25

FITTING A TAIL

A Kama Sutra classic: your lover aims to keep their heel on your forehead right until the finish. Practice makes perfect.

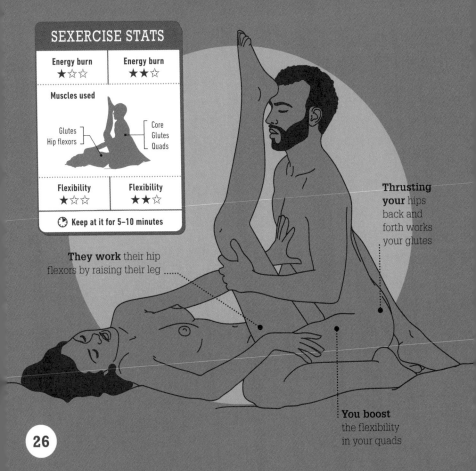

SEXERCISE STATS

Energy burn	Energy burn
★ ☆ ☆	★ ★ ☆

Muscles used

Glutes
Hip flexors

Core
Glutes
Quads

Flexibility	Flexibility
★ ☆ ☆	★ ★ ☆

🕐 Keep at it for 5–10 minutes

They work their hip flexors by raising their leg

Thrusting your hips back and forth works your glutes

You boost the flexibility in your quads

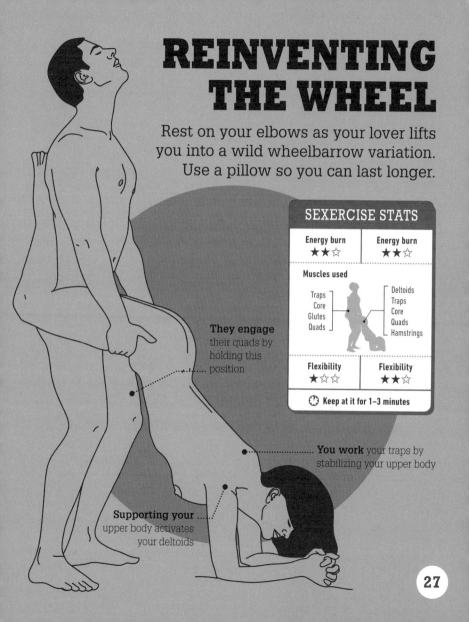

REINVENTING THE WHEEL

Rest on your elbows as your lover lifts you into a wild wheelbarrow variation. Use a pillow so you can last longer.

SEXERCISE STATS

Energy burn	Energy burn
★★☆	★★☆

Muscles used

Traps	Deltoids
Core	Traps
Glutes	Core
Quads	Quads
	Hamstrings

Flexibility	Flexibility
★☆☆	★★☆

🕓 Keep at it for 1–3 minutes

They engage their quads by holding this position

You work your traps by stabilizing your upper body

Supporting your upper body activates your deltoids

27

STRIP AND GRIP

Hold on tight as your lover thrusts at full throttle. A sofa or headboard will act as a shock absorber so you can both go wild.

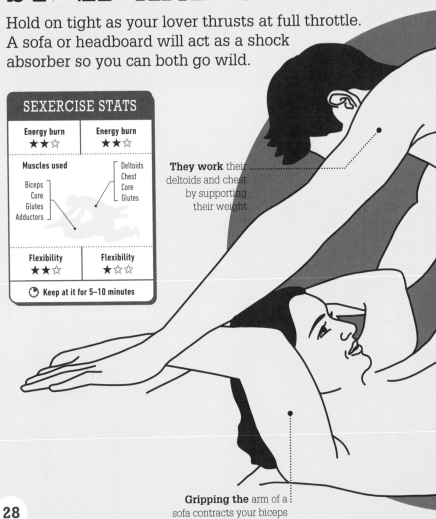

SEXERCISE STATS

Energy burn	Energy burn
★★☆	★★☆

Muscles used	
Biceps Core Glutes Adductors	Deltoids Chest Core Glutes

Flexibility	Flexibility
★★☆	★☆☆

🕐 Keep at it for 5–10 minutes

They work their deltoids and chest by supporting their weight

Gripping the arm of a sofa contracts your biceps

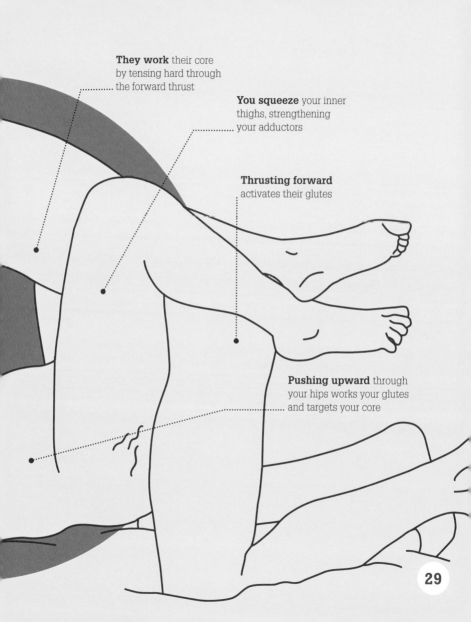

They work their core by tensing hard through the forward thrust

You squeeze your inner thighs, strengthening your adductors

Thrusting forward activates their glutes

Pushing upward through your hips works your glutes and targets your core

29

OLE DANCE

Your lover uses your leg as a pole to titillate you: they stroke, rub, or slide up and down it before sitting back on your lap and taking you for a ride.

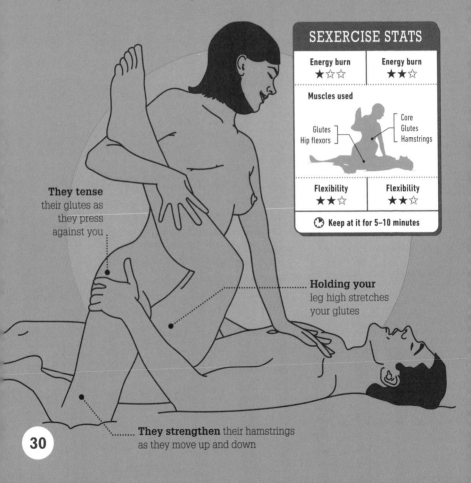

They tense their glutes as they press against you

Holding your leg high stretches your glutes

They strengthen their hamstrings as they move up and down

SEXERCISE STATS

Energy burn	Energy burn
★☆☆	★★☆

Muscles used

Glutes
Hip flexors

Core
Glutes
Hamstrings

Flexibility	Flexibility
★★☆	★★☆

🕑 **Keep at it for 5–10 minutes**

STAND TO ATTENTION

Perfect for those take-me-now moments. If you're near a wall, use your feet to push yourself on and off them.

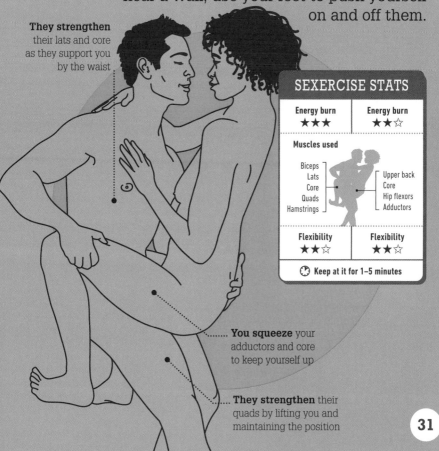

They strengthen their lats and core as they support you by the waist

SEXERCISE STATS

Energy burn	Energy burn
★★★	★★☆

Muscles used

Biceps	Upper back
Lats	Core
Core	Hip flexors
Quads	Adductors
Hamstrings	

Flexibility	Flexibility
★★☆	★★☆

🕐 Keep at it for 1–5 minutes

You squeeze your adductors and core to keep yourself up

They strengthen their quads by lifting you and maintaining the position

HEAVENLY HOLD

Take their pleasure to new heights by leaning them against a wall and licking. They can slide down to return the favor.

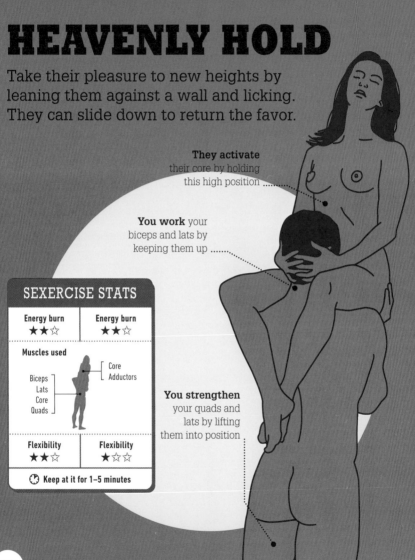

They activate their core by holding this high position ....

You work your biceps and lats by keeping them up ....

SEXERCISE STATS

Energy burn ★★☆	Energy burn ★★☆
Muscles used	Core Adductors
Biceps Lats Core Quads	
Flexibility ★★☆	Flexibility ★☆☆
🕑 Keep at it for 1–5 minutes	

You strengthen your quads and lats by lifting them into position ....

HIT THE G-SQUAT

Relish the intimacy of this sexy squat pose. It's an ideal opportunity to give special attention to your lover's chest and nipples.

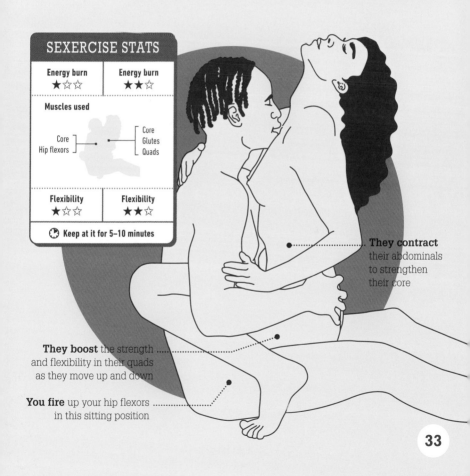

SEXERCISE STATS

Energy burn	Energy burn
★ ☆ ☆	★ ★ ☆

Muscles used

Core
Hip flexors

Core
Glutes
Quads

Flexibility	Flexibility
★ ☆ ☆	★ ★ ☆

🕐 **Keep at it for 5–10 minutes**

They contract their abdominals to strengthen their core

They boost the strength and flexibility in their quads as they move up and down

You fire up your hip flexors in this sitting position

LAVISH LEG LIFT

Your legs take center stage in this ultra-erotic position. To avoid reaching their peak too quickly, your lover can pull out and penetrate your thighs.

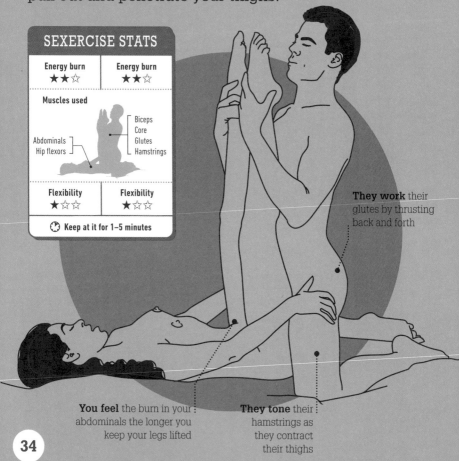

SEXERCISE STATS

Energy burn	Energy burn
★★☆	★★☆

Muscles used

Abdominals
Hip flexors

Biceps
Core
Glutes
Hamstrings

Flexibility	Flexibility
★☆☆	★☆☆

🕐 Keep at it for 1–5 minutes

They work their glutes by thrusting back and forth

You feel the burn in your abdominals the longer you keep your legs lifted

They tone their hamstrings as they contract their thighs

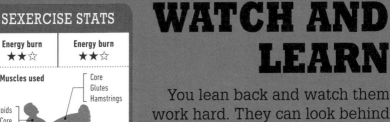

WATCH AND LEARN

You lean back and watch them work hard. They can look behind to catch sight of your pleasure.

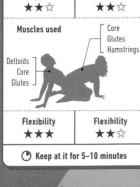

SEXERCISE STATS

Energy burn	Energy burn
★★☆	★★☆

Muscles used	
Deltoids Core Glutes	Core Glutes Hamstrings

Flexibility	Flexibility
★★★	★★☆

🕐 Keep at it for 5–10 minutes

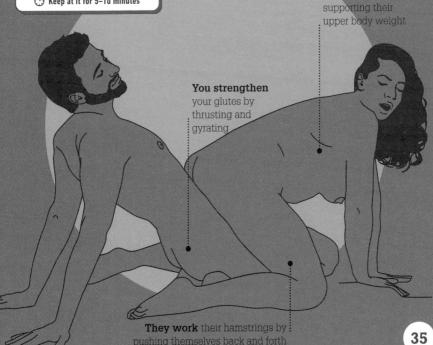

They contract their core muscles by supporting their upper body weight

You strengthen your glutes by thrusting and gyrating

They work their hamstrings by pushing themselves back and forth

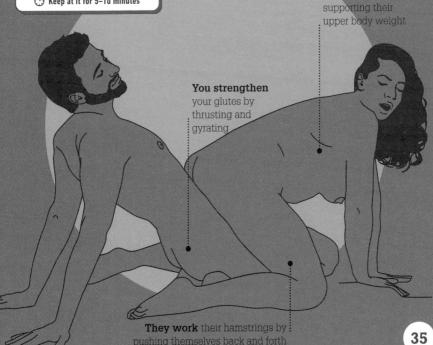

35

SEXY SUPERHERO

Let your passions take flight by lifting your legs off the floor for an intense rear-entry session. Perfect for spanking, if you've been naughty.

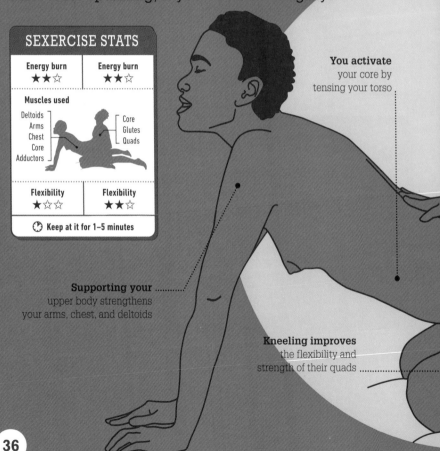

SEXERCISE STATS

Energy burn	Energy burn
★★☆	★★☆

Muscles used

Deltoids
Arms
Chest
Core
Adductors

Core
Glutes
Quads

Flexibility	Flexibility
★☆☆	★★☆

🕐 Keep at it for 1–5 minutes

You activate
your core by tensing your torso

Supporting your
upper body strengthens your arms, chest, and deltoids

Kneeling improves
the flexibility and strength of their quads

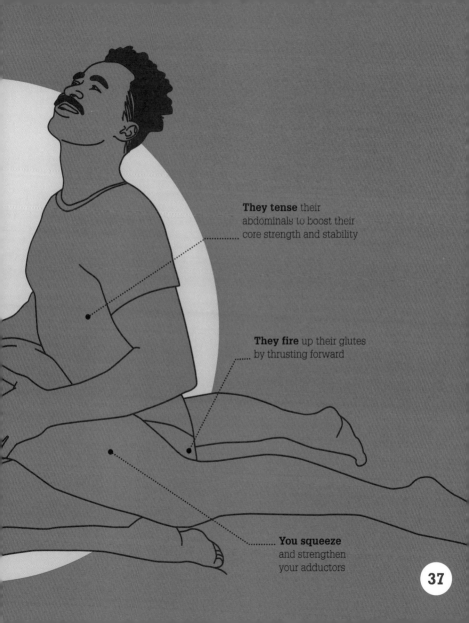

They tense their abdominals to boost their core strength and stability

They fire up their glutes by thrusting forward

You squeeze and strengthen your adductors

37

CUFF AND TUMBLE

You'll both come out on top in this erotic tussle.
Do it on the floor so you can roll around as
much as you like.

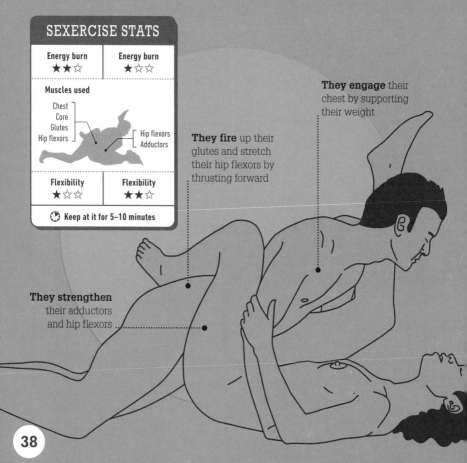

SEXERCISE STATS

Energy burn	Energy burn
★★☆	★☆☆

Muscles used

Chest
Core
Glutes
Hip flexors

Hip flexors
Adductors

Flexibility	Flexibility
★☆☆	★★☆

🕐 Keep at it for 5–10 minutes

They engage their
chest by supporting
their weight

They fire up their
glutes and stretch
their hip flexors by
thrusting forward

They strengthen
their adductors
and hip flexors

SITTING PRETTY

One partner offers their lap as a seat, then leans back to enjoy the ride. The other squeezes their thighs together to create an extra-tight fit.

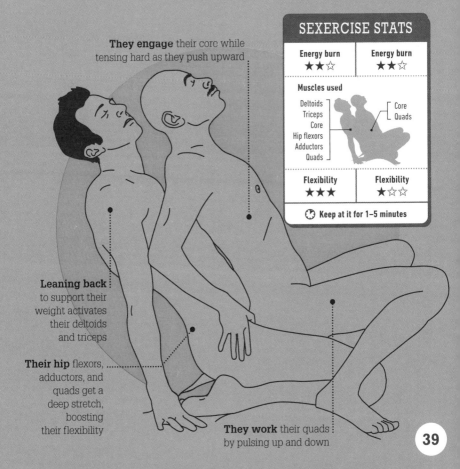

They engage their core while tensing hard as they push upward

Leaning back to support their weight activates their deltoids and triceps

Their hip flexors, adductors, and quads get a deep stretch, boosting their flexibility

They work their quads by pulsing up and down

SEXERCISE STATS

Energy burn	Energy burn
★★☆	★★☆

Muscles used

Deltoids	Core
Triceps	Quads
Core	
Hip flexors	
Adductors	
Quads	

Flexibility	Flexibility
★★★	★☆☆

🕑 Keep at it for 1–5 minutes

39

SEXUAL TENSION

Lean back and grasp each other's ankles to create this erotically taut pose. You'll both grip tightly and create delicious pangs of pleasure.

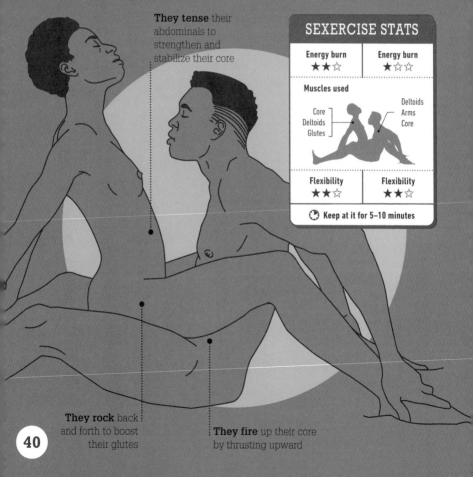

They tense their abdominals to strengthen and stabilize their core

They rock back and forth to boost their glutes

They fire up their core by thrusting upward

SEXERCISE STATS

Energy burn	Energy burn
★★☆	★☆☆

Muscles used

Core
Deltoids
Glutes

Deltoids
Arms
Core

Flexibility	Flexibility
★★☆	★★☆

🕐 Keep at it for 5–10 minutes

CORE AMOUR

Your lover's pose says, "Come and get me!" and you take them up on the challenge. Lock eyes and gaze at each other to heighten the emotional intensity.

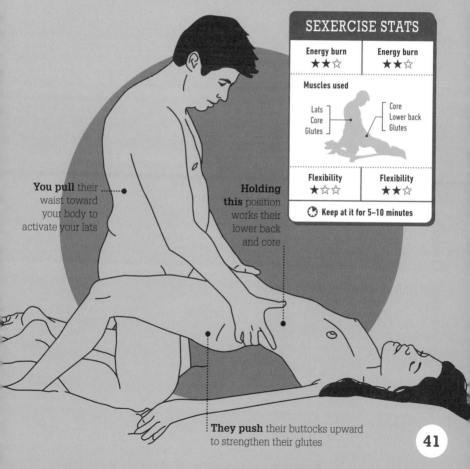

You pull their waist toward your body to activate your lats

Holding this position works their lower back and core

SEXERCISE STATS

Energy burn	Energy burn
★★☆	★★☆

Muscles used

Lats
Core
Glutes

Core
Lower back
Glutes

Flexibility	Flexibility
★☆☆	★★☆

🕐 Keep at it for 5–10 minutes

They push their buttocks upward to strengthen their glutes

41

DOUBLE ACT

Your lover sits perfectly poised on your lap, and you are enthralled by the beauty of their chest. They tease you by letting you look but not touch.

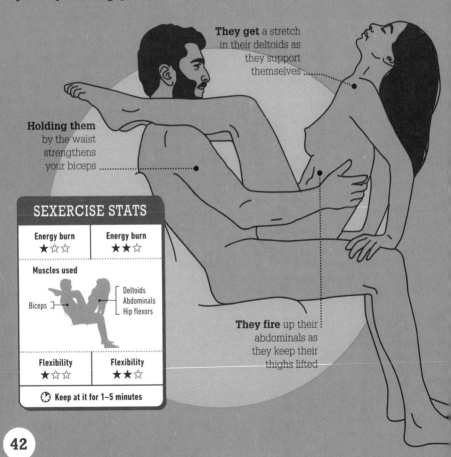

They get a stretch in their deltoids as they support themselves

Holding them by the waist strengthens your biceps

They fire up their abdominals as they keep their thighs lifted

SEXERCISE STATS

Energy burn	Energy burn
★☆☆	★★☆

Muscles used

Biceps

Deltoids
Abdominals
Hip flexors

Flexibility	Flexibility
★☆☆	★★☆

🕑 Keep at it for 1–5 minutes

FITNESS FOREPLAY

Swing your legs over your head and direct your partner to your love spot. They start slow and sensually—the more excited you get, the quicker they go.

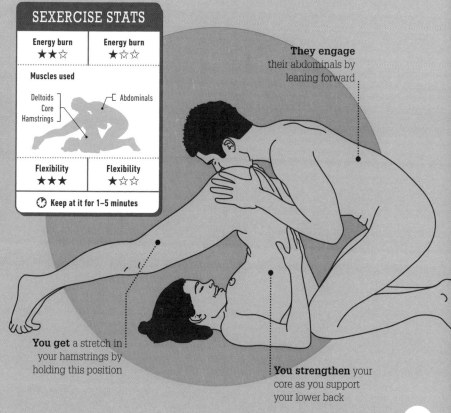

SEXERCISE STATS

Energy burn ★★☆	Energy burn ★☆☆
Muscles used	
Deltoids Core Hamstrings — Abdominals	
Flexibility ★★★	Flexibility ★☆☆
🕐 Keep at it for 1–5 minutes	

They engage their abdominals by leaning forward

You get a stretch in your hamstrings by holding this position

You strengthen your core as you support your lower back

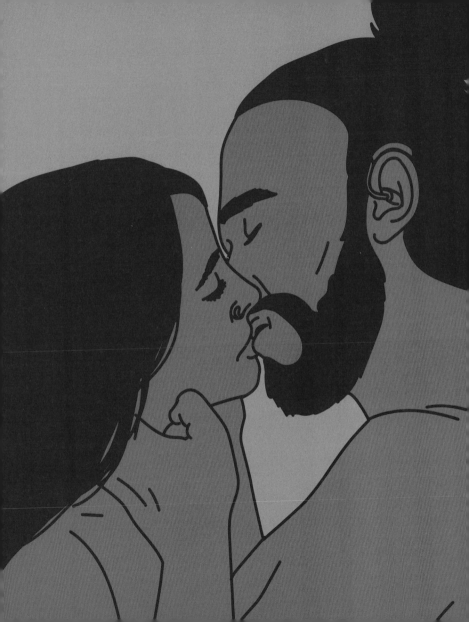

"The kiss
**IS ONE OF THE MOST
POWERFUL
STIMULANTS TO THE
WORK OF LOVE "**

THE PERFUMED GARDEN

LAP IT UP

The seated partner can thrust deeply or grind in circles to bring the other to orgasm. The hot view of bare buttocks is a cheeky bonus.

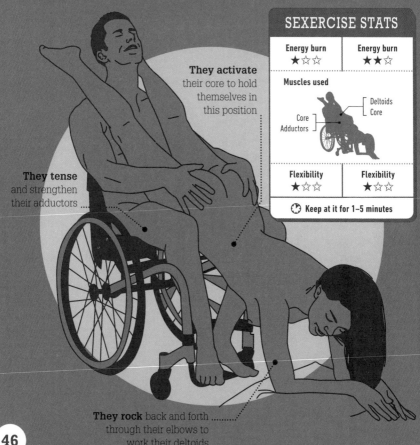

They activate their core to hold themselves in this position

They tense and strengthen their adductors

They rock back and forth through their elbows to work their deltoids

SEXERCISE STATS

Energy burn	Energy burn
★☆☆	★★☆

Muscles used

Deltoids
Core
Core
Adductors

Flexibility	Flexibility
★☆☆	★☆☆

🕐 Keep at it for 1–5 minutes

LUSTFUL LEG PRESS

This intimate position creates extra-deep penetration, so start gently, then let your lust run wild.

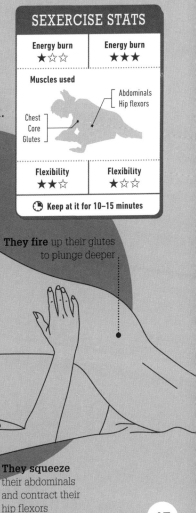

Supporting their weight targets their chest and core

They fire up their glutes to plunge deeper

They squeeze their abdominals and contract their hip flexors

47

ROUGH DIAMOND

Your lover stretches their legs wide, and you ease their feet together to form a divine diamond. Their hands are free to bring themselves to a shuddering orgasm.

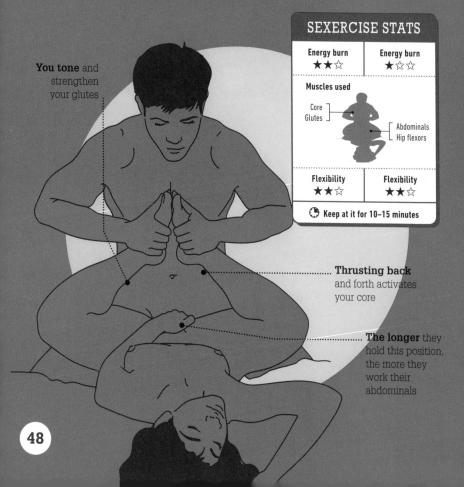

You tone and strengthen your glutes

SEXERCISE STATS

Energy burn	Energy burn
★★☆	★☆☆

Muscles used

Core
Glutes

Abdominals
Hip flexors

Flexibility	Flexibility
★★☆	★★☆

🕐 **Keep at it for 10–15 minutes**

Thrusting back and forth activates your core

The longer they hold this position, the more they work their abdominals

SLIPPERY WHEN WET

You squeeze your thighs together tightly while your lover thrusts between them. Cover yourselves in oil to make it super slippery and sensual.

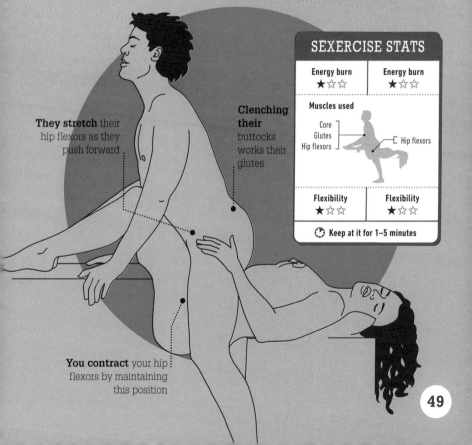

They stretch their hip flexors as they push forward

Clenching their buttocks works their glutes

You contract your hip flexors by maintaining this position

SEXERCISE STATS

Energy burn	Energy burn
★☆☆	★☆☆

Muscles used

Core
Glutes
Hip flexors

Hip flexors

Flexibility	Flexibility
★☆☆	★☆☆

🕑 Keep at it for 1–5 minutes

PRIMAL INSTINCTS

A sumptuously simple pose that brings you back to basics. Get down on all fours and hump your way to happiness.

Rocking back and forth engages your glutes

Pushing their body backward works their hamstrings

They thrust back and forth with their hips to activate their glutes

50

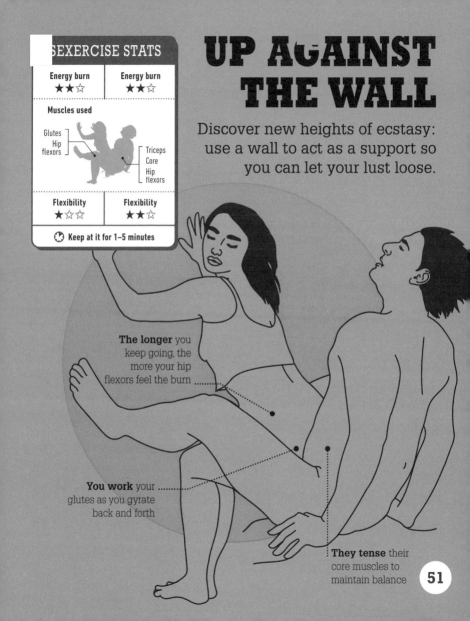

EXERCISE STATS

Energy burn	Energy burn
★★☆	★★☆

Muscles used

Glutes
Hip flexors

Triceps
Core
Hip flexors

Flexibility	Flexibility
★☆☆	★★☆

🕓 Keep at it for 1–5 minutes

UP AGAINST THE WALL

Discover new heights of ecstasy: use a wall to act as a support so you can let your lust loose.

The longer you keep going, the more your hip flexors feel the burn

You work your glutes as you gyrate back and forth

They tense their core muscles to maintain balance

ENTER THE LION'S DEN

For seriously hot and voracious sex, your partner lies back with their hips high, and you lean in lustfully.

SEXERCISE STATS

Energy burn	Energy burn
★★☆	★★☆

Muscles used

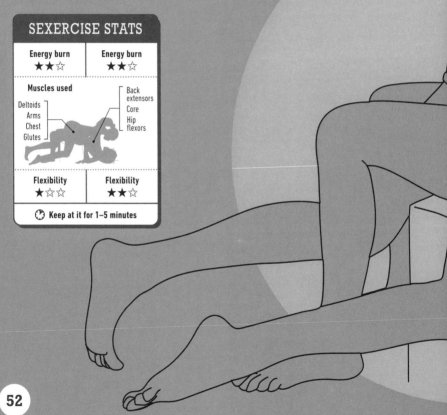

Deltoids
Arms
Chest
Glutes

Back extensors
Core
Hip flexors

Flexibility	Flexibility
★☆☆	★★☆

🕐 Keep at it for 1–5 minutes

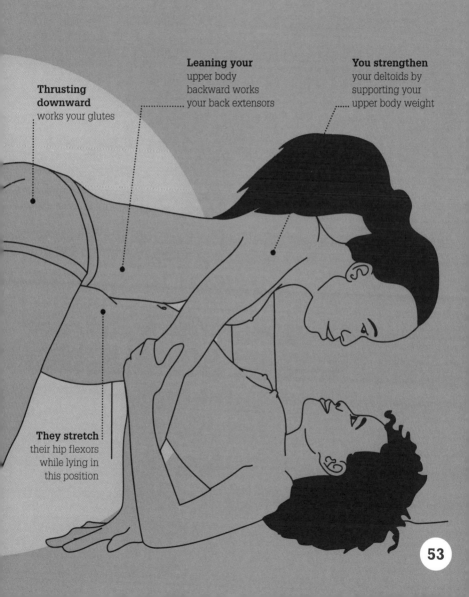

Thrusting downward works your glutes

Leaning your upper body backward works your back extensors

You strengthen your deltoids by supporting your upper body weight

They stretch their hip flexors while lying in this position

53

LEAN OF FAITH

You grip each other's wrists, lean back, then push and pull until the tension reaches breaking point.

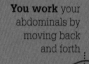
You work your abdominals by moving back and forth

Drawing you toward them strengthens their lats

They feel the burn in their core as they keep themselves stable

SEXERCISE STATS

Energy burn	Energy burn
★★☆	★☆☆

Muscles used

Glutes
Core

Glutes
Core

Flexibility	Flexibility
★☆☆	★☆☆

🕑 Keep at it for 5–10 minutes

You bow down at your lover's feet and show your adoration. They clasp your buttocks and enjoy the view.

Holding this position works your glutes

You build core stability by keeping yourself bent over

Thrusting upward through their hips activates their glutes

DIVE IN DEEP

Your partner leans forward to let you plunge in. You can thrust deeply, unleashing irresistible shivers of pleasure.

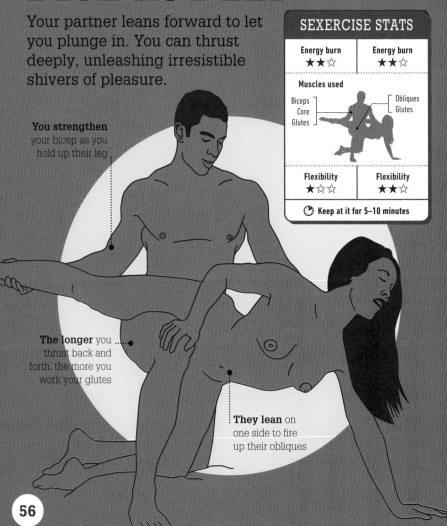

You strengthen your bicep as you hold up their leg

The longer you thrust back and forth, the more you work your glutes

They lean on one side to fire up their obliques

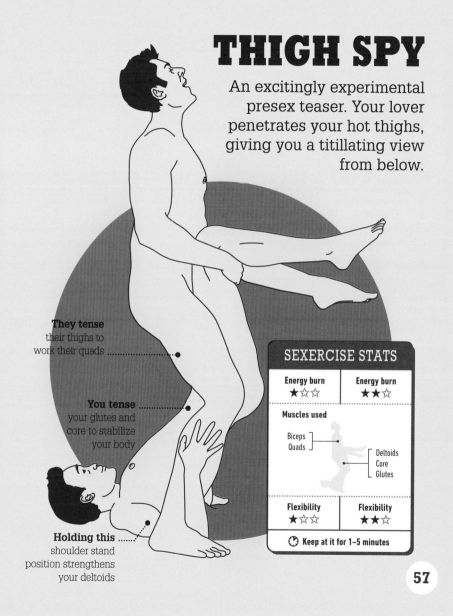

THIGH SPY

An excitingly experimental presex teaser. Your lover penetrates your hot thighs, giving you a titillating view from below.

They tense their thighs to work their quads

You tense your glutes and core to stabilize your body

Holding this shoulder stand position strengthens your deltoids

SEXERCISE STATS

Energy burn	Energy burn
★☆☆	★★☆

Muscles used

Biceps
Quads

Deltoids
Core
Glutes

Flexibility	Flexibility
★☆☆	★★☆

⏱ Keep at it for 1–5 minutes

57

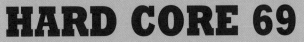

HARD CORE 69

An undisputed classic with a head-turning twist: pleasure each other for as long as you can, then finish on the floor.

They fire up their core to hold themselves upside down ....

They can turn the heat up in their biceps by holding their partner for as long as they can

SEXERCISE STATS

Energy burn	Energy burn
★★☆	★★☆

Muscles used

Biceps
Chest
Core

Biceps
Chest
Core
Quads
Hamstrings

Flexibility	Flexibility
★☆☆	★☆☆

🕐 Keep at it for 1–5 minutes

They push hard through their quads and hamstrings to lift their partner

BALANCING ACT

Clasp your arms around each other and bounce gently in this dirty double squat. It guarantees plenty of hot and sweaty skin-on-skin action.

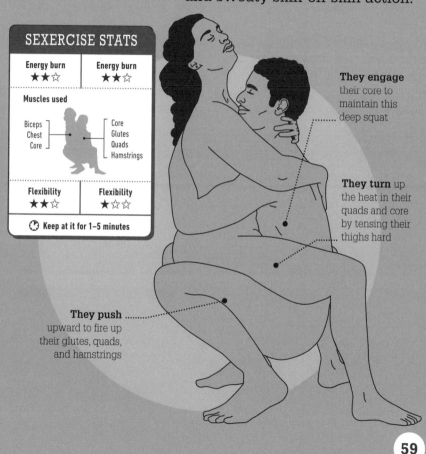

SEXERCISE STATS

Energy burn	Energy burn
★★☆	★★☆

Muscles used

Biceps
Chest
Core

Core
Glutes
Quads
Hamstrings

Flexibility	Flexibility
★★☆	★☆☆

🕐 Keep at it for 1–5 minutes

They engage their core to maintain this deep squat

They turn up the heat in their quads and core by tensing their thighs hard

They push upward to fire up their glutes, quads, and hamstrings

TARGET PRACTICE

You are the bow in this elegant position, and your arrow is on target. Lifting your lover's leg lets you slide in farther for deep penetration.

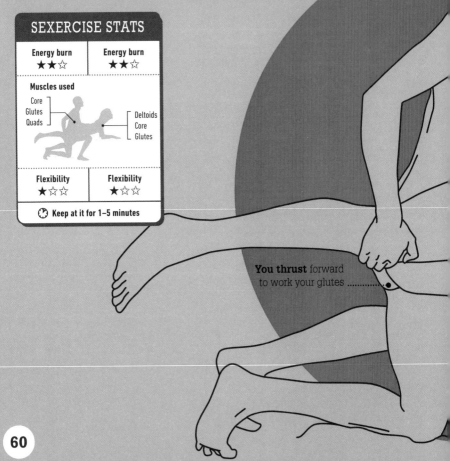

SEXERCISE STATS

Energy burn ★★☆	Energy burn ★★☆

Muscles used

Core
Glutes
Quads

Deltoids
Core
Glutes

Flexibility ★☆☆	Flexibility ★☆☆

🕐 Keep at it for 1–5 minutes

You thrust forward to work your glutes

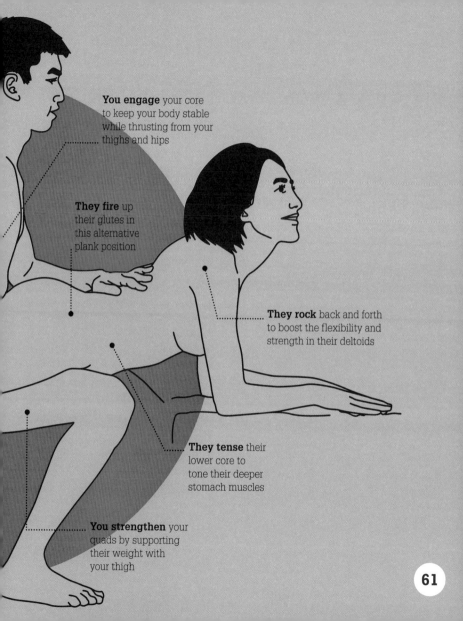

You engage your core to keep your body stable while thrusting from your thighs and hips

They fire up their glutes in this alternative plank position

They rock back and forth to boost the flexibility and strength in their deltoids

They tense their lower core to tone their deeper stomach muscles

You strengthen your quads by supporting their weight with your thigh

61

ROW YOUR BOAT

You both slot in, then rock back and forth. Let yourselves be carried along by the currents of your passion.

They work their abdominals as they reach forward

They contract their hip flexors and core as they hold this pose

Rocking back and forth works their hip flexors

KNEELING NUDE

Help your partner up into a hot half-shoulderstand.
They can bring their knees down to their chest
to let you enter more deeply.

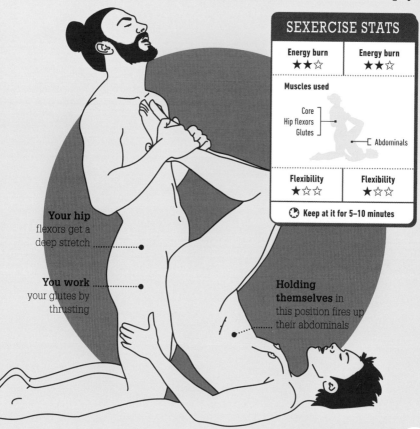

Your hip
flexors get a
deep stretch

You work
your glutes by
thrusting

**Holding
themselves** in
this position fires up
their abdominals

SEXERCISE STATS

Energy burn	Energy burn
★★☆	★★☆

Muscles used

Core
Hip flexors
Glutes
Abdominals

Flexibility	Flexibility
★☆☆	★☆☆

🕑 **Keep at it for 5–10 minutes**

DERRIÈRE DELIGHT

Enjoy this exotic angle as your lover swings their buttocks back and forth to give you a super-hot view.

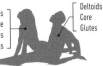
They rock back and forth to work their hamstrings

They support their weight with their deltoids

You strengthen your glutes by tensing your buttocks as you thrust forward

TWINKLE TOES

The feeling of your legs pressed against your partner's upper body gets them going and makes you feel like a superstar.

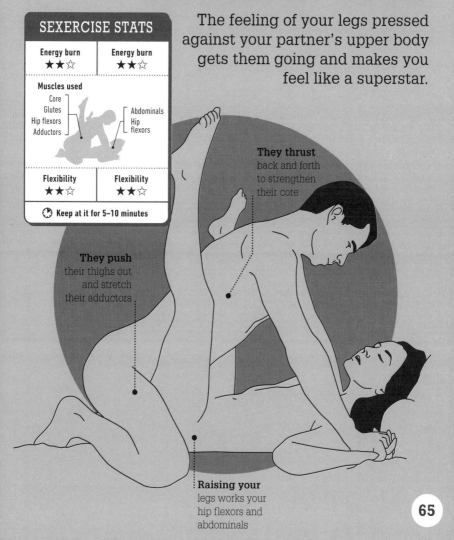

They thrust back and forth to strengthen their core

They push their thighs out and stretch their adductors

Raising your legs works your hip flexors and abdominals

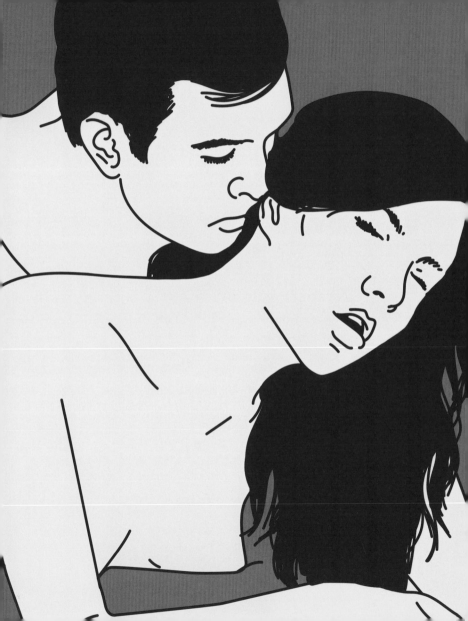

"*You should feel* **THE WHOLE** OF THEIR BODY **WITH YOUR HANDS,** AND KISS THEM *all over*"

THE KAMA SUTRA

STANDING ROOM ONLY

A naughty knee-trembler: you both step one foot forward and unleash your lust.

SEXERCISE STATS

Energy burn	Energy burn
★★☆	★★☆

Muscles used

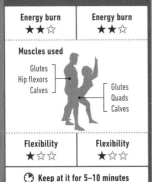

Glutes
Hip flexors
Calves

Glutes
Quads
Calves

Flexibility	Flexibility
★☆☆	★☆☆

🕐 Keep at it for 5–10 minutes

Thrusting their hips fires up their glutes

They stretch the hip flexors in their back thigh

They boost the flexibility in their calves

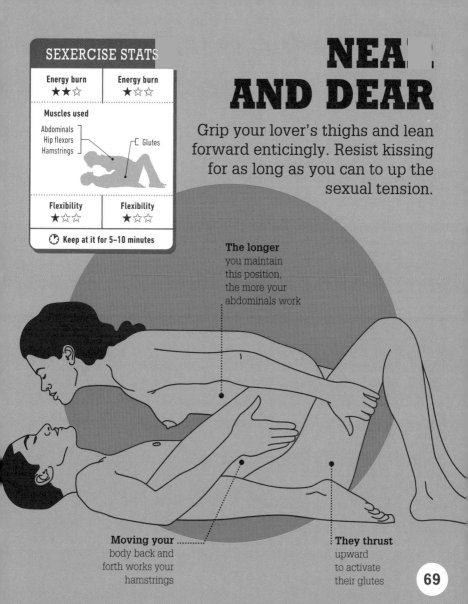

Energy burn	Energy burn
★★☆	★☆☆

Muscles used

Abdominals
Hip flexors
Hamstrings

⌐ Glutes

Flexibility	Flexibility
★☆☆	★☆☆

🕓 Keep it for 5–10 minutes

NEAR AND DEAR

Grip your lover's thighs and lean forward enticingly. Resist kissing for as long as you can to up the sexual tension.

The longer you maintain this position, the more your abdominals work

Moving your body back and forth works your hamstrings

They thrust upward to activate their glutes

■EART-STOP■ING HOLD

Your lover sweeps you away in their arms and swings you up against a wall.

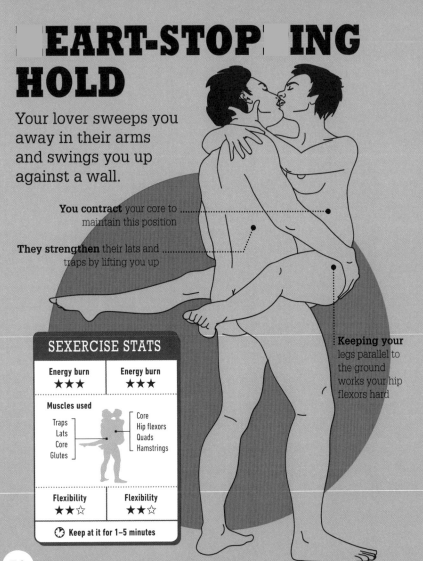

You contract your core to maintain this position

They strengthen their lats and traps by lifting you up

Keeping your legs parallel to the ground works your hip flexors hard

SEXERCISE STATS

Energy burn	Energy burn
★★★	★★★

Muscles used

Traps
Lats
Core
Glutes

Core
Hip flexors
Quads
Hamstrings

Flexibility	Flexibility
★★☆	★★☆

🕐 **Keep at it for 1–5 minutes**

SITTING TIGHT

Seal the intimacy of this compact position with a lingering kiss. You pull your partner in close until their chest presses against their thighs.

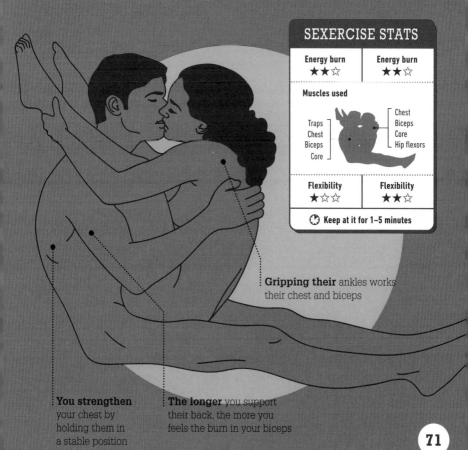

SEXERCISE STATS

Energy burn	Energy burn
★★☆	★★☆

Muscles used

Traps
Chest
Biceps
Core

Chest
Biceps
Core
Hip flexors

Flexibility	Flexibility
★☆☆	★★☆

🕐 Keep at it for 1–5 minutes

Gripping their ankles works their chest and biceps

You strengthen your chest by holding them in a stable position

The longer you support their back, the more you feels the burn in your biceps

PRESS-UP PLEASURE

Twirl your tongue and make your lover tremble with desire. They hold themselves up until they can't take it anymore.

They feel the burn in their arms and deltoids

They work their core strength and stability

You contract your biceps by holding their thighs

72

LAP OF LUXURY

Embrace hungrily and shower each other with kisses and caresses. When you're both burning with desire, you can let your lover in.

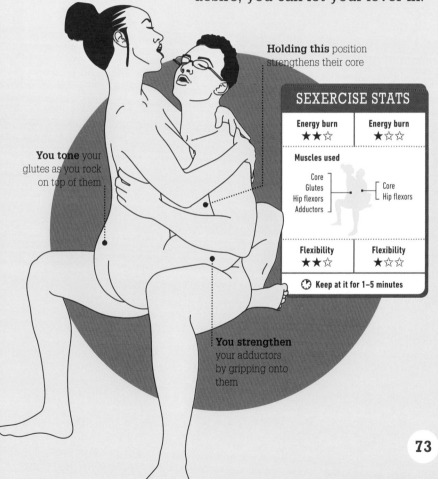

Holding this position strengthens their core

You tone your glutes as you rock on top of them

You strengthen your adductors by gripping onto them

SEXERCISE STATS

Energy burn	Energy burn
★★☆	★☆☆

Muscles used

Core
Glutes
Hip flexors
Adductors

Core
Hip flexors

Flexibility	Flexibility
★★☆	★☆☆

🕑 **Keep at it for 1–5 minutes**

AT FULL THRUST

Your partner pumps like a steam train while you give directions from the rear and relish the sight of their buttocks.

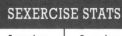
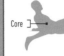
Contract your deep core muscles to hold this pose

They work their arms and deltoids as they rock back and forth

They squeeze their adductors to maintain contact with your body

74

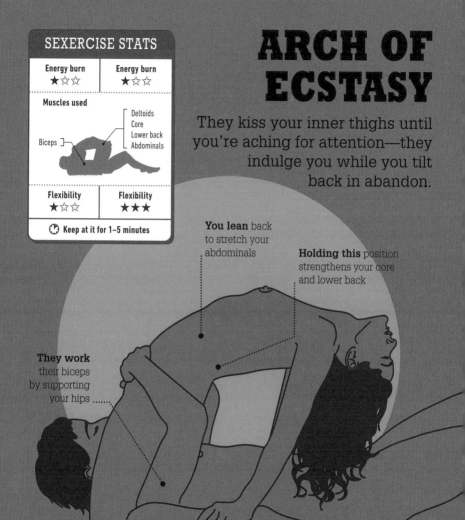

ARCH OF ECSTASY

They kiss your inner thighs until you're aching for attention—they indulge you while you tilt back in abandon.

SEXERCISE STATS

Energy burn	Energy burn
★☆☆	★☆☆

Muscles used

Biceps

Deltoids
Core
Lower back
Abdominals

Flexibility	Flexibility
★☆☆	★★★

🕑 Keep at it for 1–5 minutes

You lean back to stretch your abdominals

Holding this position strengthens your core and lower back

They work their biceps by supporting your hips

DOWN TO BUSINESS

A rear-entry position that's sure to shake up your sex life. You tuck up tightly and let your lover take control.

They work their glutes by thrusting

Holding this position strengthens your deltoids

SEXERCISE STATS

Energy burn	Energy burn
★★★	★☆☆

Muscles used

Deltoids
Hamstrings
Abdominals

Biceps
Lats
Glutes

Flexibility	Flexibility
★★☆	★☆☆

🕐 Keep at it for 1–5 minutes

You test your abdominal power and strength

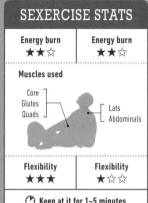

SEXERCISE STATS

Energy burn	Energy burn
★★☆	★★☆
Muscles used	
Core Glutes Quads — Lats Abdominals	
Flexibility	Flexibility
★★★	★☆☆
🕑 Keep at it for 1–5 minutes	

ATTENTION GRABBING

When you can't keep your hands off each other, clasp hold and seesaw your way to sexual satisfaction.

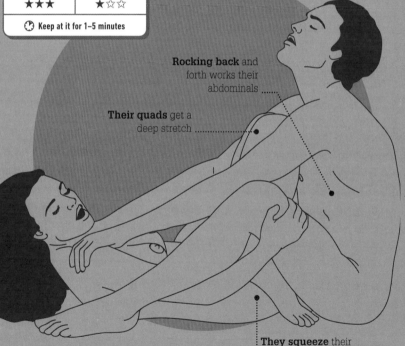

Rocking back and forth works their abdominals ......

Their quads get a deep stretch ....

They squeeze their glutes and core to hold this position

THREE-LEGGED DOG

A sizzling-hot standing position that is easier than it looks: you can try lifting both your partner's legs to take it up a notch.

SEXERCISE STATS

Energy burn	Energy burn
★★☆	★★☆

Muscles used	
Lats Glutes Hip flexors	Deltoids Core Hip flexors Glutes Quads Hamstrings

Flexibility	Flexibility
★☆☆	★★☆

🕑 Keep at it for 1–5 minutes

They get a deep stretch in their hip flexors

You thrust forward to stretch your hip flexors

This position tests the strength in their quads and hamstrings as they balance on one leg

78

SIDESADDLE

Start by spooning, then you straddle your lover's legs and reach forward to clasp their calves. Rolling onto your back unleashes even more divine sensations.

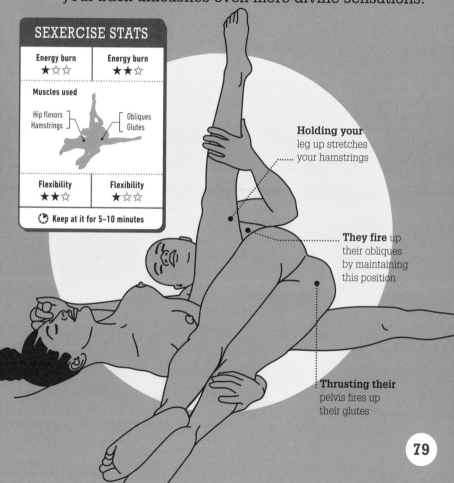

SEXERCISE STATS

Energy burn	Energy burn
★☆☆	★★☆

Muscles used

Hip flexors
Hamstrings

Obliques
Glutes

Flexibility	Flexibility
★★☆	★☆☆

🕒 Keep at it for 5–10 minutes

Holding your leg up stretches your hamstrings

They fire up their obliques by maintaining this position

Thrusting their pelvis fires up their glutes

FEET-UP FELLATIO

Your lover holds a shoulder stand while you use your mouth to get them going. They get the bonus view of your beautiful bouncing body.

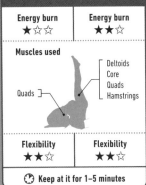

SEXERCISE STATS

Energy burn ★☆☆	Energy burn ★★☆
Muscles used Quads]	[Deltoids Core Quads Hamstrings
Flexibility ★★☆	Flexibility ★★☆

🕑 Keep at it for 1–5 minutes

They fire up their quads and hamstrings to hold up their legs

The longer they hold this position, the more they strengthen their core

You feel the stretch in your quads as you sit in this position

LYING LOW

For deliciously lazy lovemaking, your partner lies back while you thrust gently. Use your hand to bring them to a breathtaking climax.

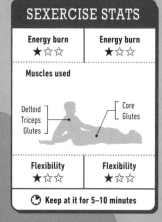

SEXERCISE STATS

Energy burn	Energy burn
★☆☆	★☆☆

Muscles used

Deltoid
Triceps
Glutes

Core
Glutes

Flexibility	Flexibility
★☆☆	★☆☆

🕑 Keep at it for 5–10 minutes

They work their core by squeezing their abdominals

Rocking toward you contracts their glutes

You thrust upward to work your glutes

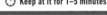

Lock your legs seductively around your partner's torso and pull them toward you. They lean over you to thrust powerfully.

They strengthen their biceps by supporting your weight

Gripping their torso with your thighs activates your adductors

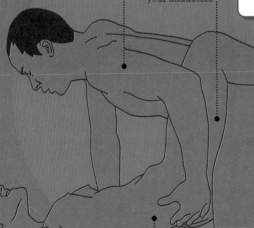

You squeeze your buttocks and push upward to work your core

VERTICAL LOVE LIFT

Support your love against a wall and let your passion loose. Ideal for quenching your lust in unusual places.

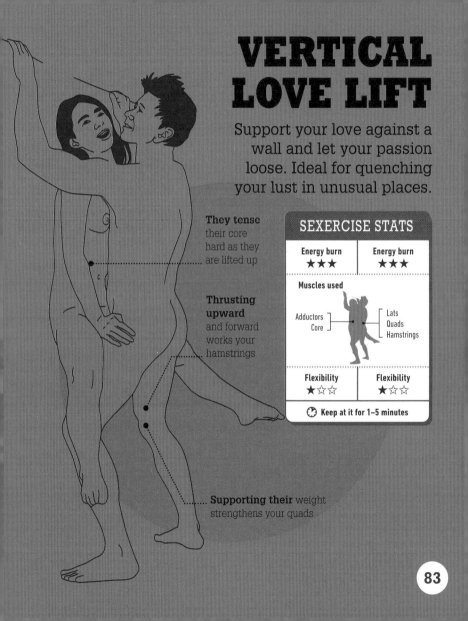

They tense their core hard as they are lifted up

Thrusting upward and forward works your hamstrings

Supporting their weight strengthens your quads

SEXERCISE STATS

Energy burn	Energy burn
★★★	★★★

Muscles used

Adductors
Core

Lats
Quads
Hamstrings

Flexibility	Flexibility
★☆☆	★☆☆

🕐 Keep at it for 1–5 minutes

BEND AND BLOW

Use your hands, lips, and tongue to explore your lover's erogenous zones while they watch the action from a novel angle.

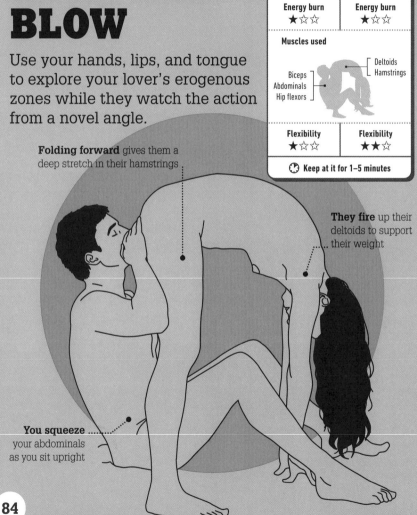

Folding forward gives them a deep stretch in their hamstrings

They fire up their deltoids to support their weight

You squeeze your abdominals as you sit upright

84

LOCK THEM IN

Cross your ankles behind your partner to pull them in deeper. Pressing their perineum with your heel gives them extra sparks of bliss.

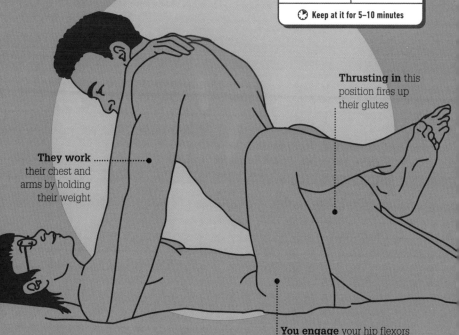

Thrusting in this position fires up their glutes

They work their chest and arms by holding their weight

You engage your hip flexors maintaining this position

SEESAW TO SATISFACTION

Graduate to this position from a 69 by sliding forward so that your lover can enter you. You can't see each other, so be sure to communicate your enjoyment loudly.

You squeeze your hamstrings to keep your feet in position

The longer you keep at it, the harder you work your abdominals and hip flexors

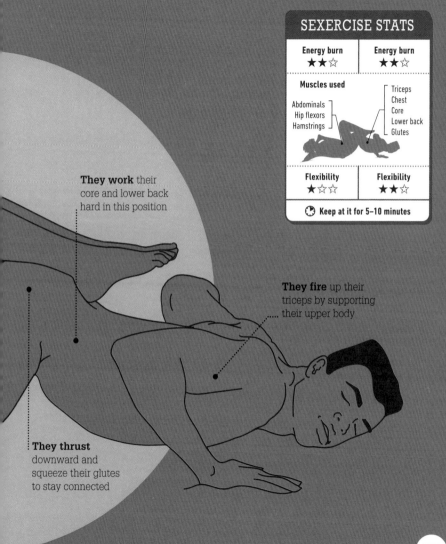

SEXERCISE STATS

Energy burn	Energy burn
★★☆	★★☆

Muscles used

Abdominals
Hip flexors
Hamstrings

Triceps
Chest
Core
Lower back
Glutes

Flexibility	Flexibility
★☆☆	★★☆

🕐 Keep at it for 5–10 minutes

They work their core and lower back hard in this position

They fire up their triceps by supporting their upper body

They thrust downward and squeeze their glutes to stay connected

87

CHEEK TO CHEEK

Face each other and press your buttocks together. Hold your partner firmly as they lean back and lose themselves to pleasure.

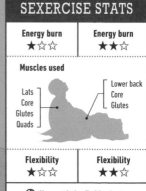

SEXERCISE STATS

Energy burn	Energy burn
★☆☆	★★☆

Muscles used

Lats
Core
Glutes
Quads

Lower back
Core
Glutes

Flexibility	Flexibility
★☆☆	★★☆

⏱ Keep at it for 5–10 minutes

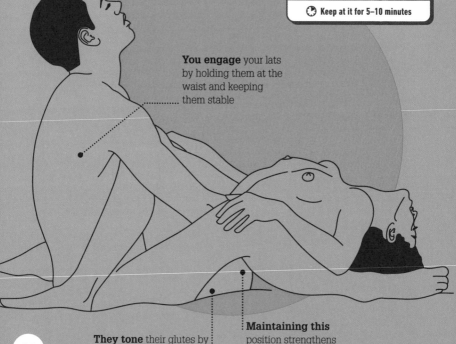

You engage your lats by holding them at the waist and keeping them stable

They tone their glutes by squeezing against you

Maintaining this position strengthens their lower back

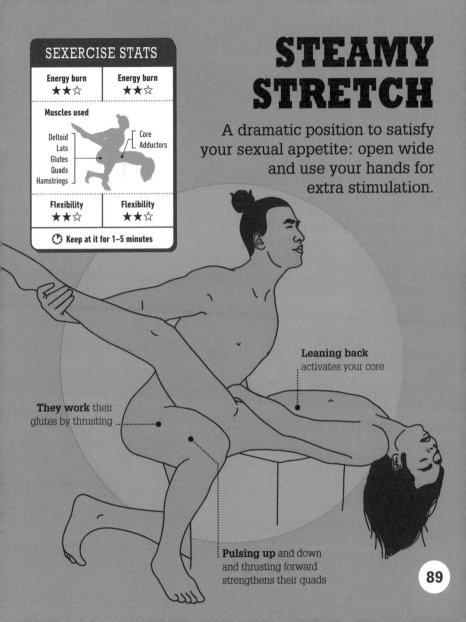

SEXERCISE STATS

Energy burn ★★☆	Energy burn ★★☆
Muscles used	
Deltoid Lats Glutes Quads Hamstrings	Core Adductors
Flexibility ★★☆	Flexibility ★★☆
🕐 Keep at it for 1–5 minutes	

STEAMY STRETCH

A dramatic position to satisfy your sexual appetite: open wide and use your hands for extra stimulation.

Leaning back activates your core

They work their glutes by thrusting

Pulsing up and down and thrusting forward strengthens their quads

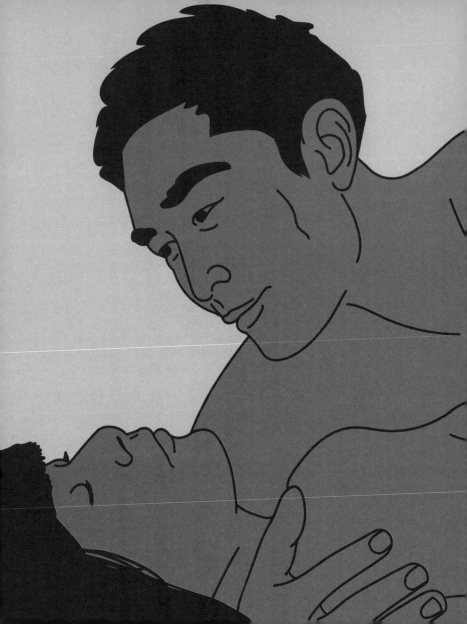

"*As one soul*
IN A SINGLE BODY
THEY SHALL BE
happy
IN THIS WORLD"

THE ANANGA RANGA

INVERTED WHEELBARROW

All the sauciness of the rear-entry position, but with added eye contact. Your partner cradles you in their arms so you feel lovingly held.

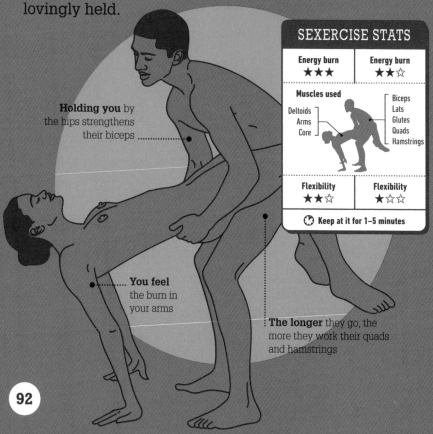

Holding you by the hips strengthens their biceps

You feel the burn in your arms

The longer they go, the more they work their quads and hamstrings

SEXERCISE STATS

Energy burn	Energy burn
★★★	★★☆

Muscles used

Deltoids
Arms
Core

Biceps
Lats
Glutes
Quads
Hamstrings

Flexibility	Flexibility
★★☆	★☆☆

🕑 **Keep at it for 1–5 minutes**

BACK-SEAT DRIVER

The fact that you don't face each other in this position gives it an extra edge of naughtiness. Plus, it's perfect for g-spot stimulation.

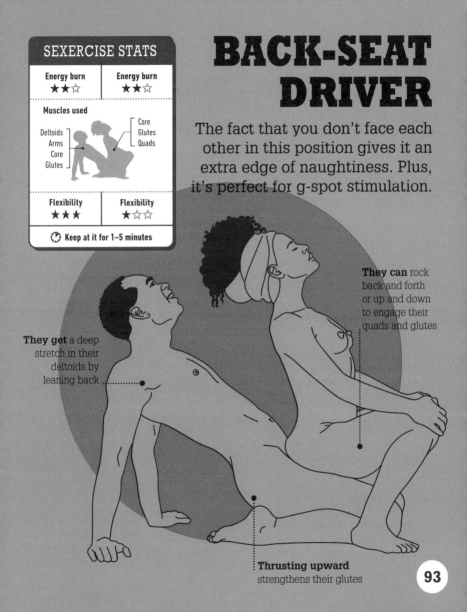

They can rock back and forth or up and down to engage their quads and glutes

They get a deep stretch in their deltoids by leaning back

Thrusting upward strengthens their glutes

BEND OVER BACKWARD

You are a gorgeous gymnast and they are the judge. They give you 10 out of 10 for a spectacular performance.

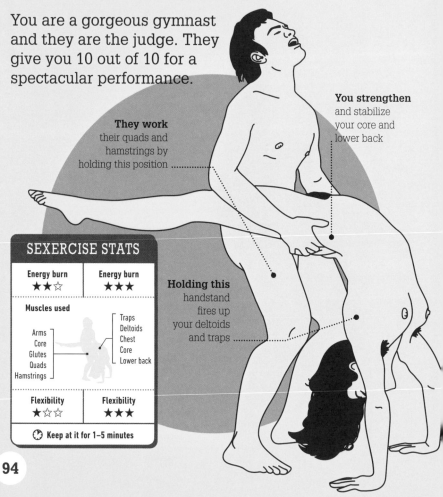

They work their quads and hamstrings by holding this position

You strengthen and stabilize your core and lower back

Holding this handstand fires up your deltoids and traps

SEXERCISE STATS

Energy burn	Energy burn
★★☆	★★★

Muscles used

Arms
Core
Glutes
Quads
Hamstrings

- Traps
- Deltoids
- Chest
- Core
- Lower back

Flexibility	Flexibility
★☆☆	★★★

🕐 Keep at it for 1–5 minutes

NAVEL GAZING

Look unwaveringly into your lover's eyes as you pleasure them. They pull you in with their foot and keep you there for as long as they like.

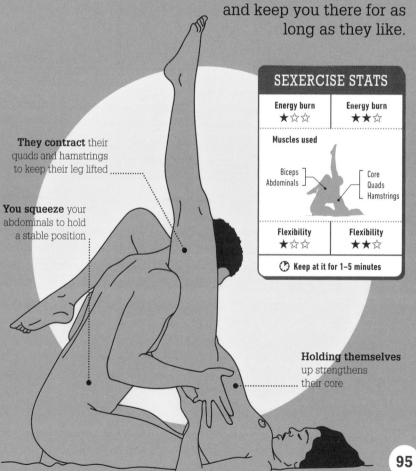

They contract their quads and hamstrings to keep their leg lifted

You squeeze your abdominals to hold a stable position

Holding themselves up strengthens their core

SEXERCISE STATS

Energy burn	Energy burn
★☆☆	★★☆

Muscles used

Biceps
Abdominals

Core
Quads
Hamstrings

Flexibility	Flexibility
★☆☆	★★☆

🕑 Keep at it for 1–5 minutes

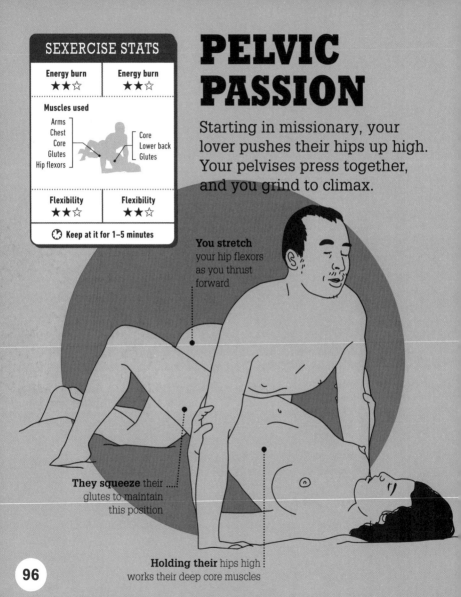

SEXERCISE STATS

Energy burn	Energy burn
★★☆	★★☆

Muscles used

Arms
Chest
Core
Glutes
Hip flexors

Core
Lower back
Glutes

Flexibility	Flexibility
★★☆	★★☆

🕐 Keep at it for 1–5 minutes

PELVIC PASSION

Starting in missionary, your lover pushes their hips up high. Your pelvises press together, and you grind to climax.

You stretch your hip flexors as you thrust forward

They squeeze their glutes to maintain this position

Holding their hips high works their deep core muscles

BACK STROKE

Ride your lover until you both reach the edge. They can make you shiver with pleasure by caressing your back or fondling your chest lovingly from behind.

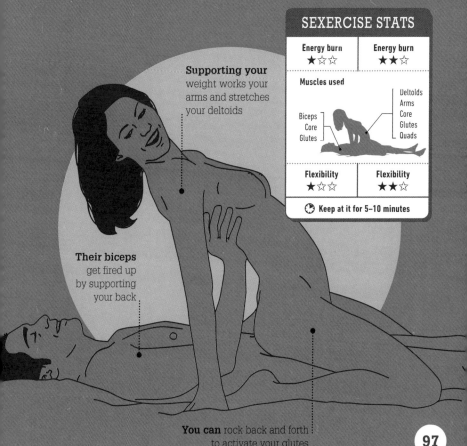

Supporting your weight works your arms and stretches your deltoids

Their biceps get fired up by supporting your back

You can rock back and forth to activate your glutes

SEXERCISE STATS

Energy burn	Energy burn
★☆☆	★★☆

Muscles used

Biceps
Core
Glutes

Deltoids
Arms
Core
Glutes
Quads

Flexibility	Flexibility
★☆☆	★★☆

🕑 **Keep at it for 5–10 minutes**

SEXY CYCLIST

Your thighs are the handlebars and your lover saddles up for a ride. They feel you grip and squeeze both inside and out.

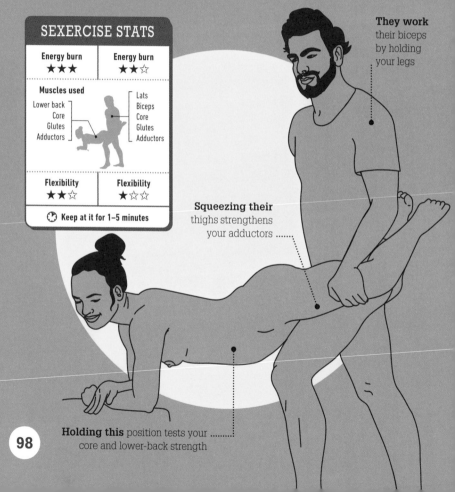

SEXERCISE STATS

Energy burn	Energy burn
★★★	★★☆

Muscles used

Lower back Core Glutes Adductors	Lats Biceps Core Glutes Adductors

Flexibility	Flexibility
★★☆	★☆☆

🕐 Keep at it for 1–5 minutes

They work their biceps by holding your legs

Squeezing their thighs strengthens your adductors

Holding this position tests your core and lower-back strength

FLIRTY FLAMINGOS

You both lift one leg in this standing pose. Clasp each other tight and try not to topple over.

Holding this position tests their core stability and balance

They strengthen their quads and hamstrings by standing on one leg

They rise onto their toes to work their calves

SEXERCISE STATS

Energy burn ★★☆	Energy burn ★★☆
Muscles used	
Core Hip flexors Calves	Core Quads Hamstrings
Flexibility ★★☆	Flexibility ★☆☆
🕐 Keep at it for 1–5 minutes	

99

CHEEKY CHALLENGE

Explore the realms of possibility by bending over and rubbing cheeks. Then turn around and go back to basics.

SEXERCISE STATS

Energy burn ★★☆	Energy burn ★★☆
Muscles used	Deltoids / Abdominals / Hamstrings
Deltoids / Abdominals	
Flexibility ★★☆	**Flexibility** ★★☆

🕐 Keep at it for 1–5 minutes

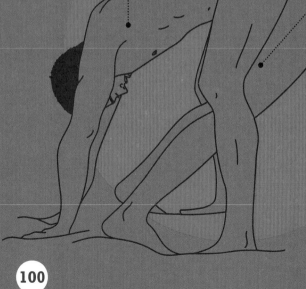

Holding this position strengthens your deltoids

They get a deep stretch in their hamstrings

Maintaining this forward fold works their abdominals

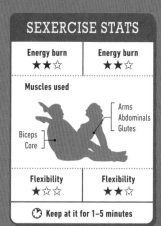
CAUGHT IN A TRAP

Grip your partner's ankles and trap them between your legs. They can add extra sparks by biting or kissing your calves.

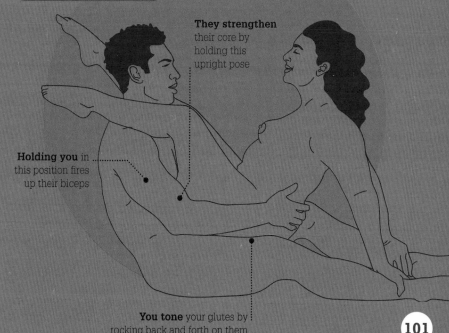

They strengthen their core by holding this upright pose

Holding you in this position fires up their biceps

You tone your glutes by rocking back and forth on them

CLOSE AND COMPACT

Whisper sweet nothings to each other or decide to talk dirty. You can keep one foot on the floor to allow extra-deep penetration.

SEXERCISE STATS

Energy burn	Energy burn
★★☆	★★☆

Muscles used

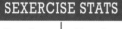

Core Glutes Hip flexors	Core Hip flexors Calves

Flexibility	Flexibility
★★☆	★★☆

🕐 **Keep at it for 1–5 minutes**

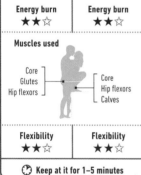

The longer you maintain this position, the more you work your core

They strengthen their glutes by thrusting forward with their pelvis

You push up through your toes to activate your calves

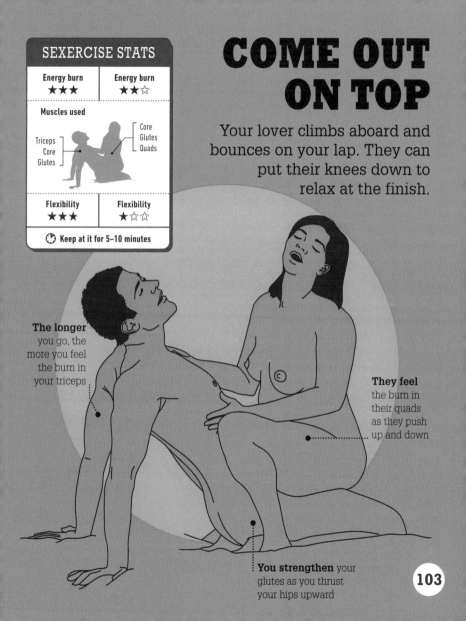

COME OUT ON TOP

Your lover climbs aboard and bounces on your lap. They can put their knees down to relax at the finish.

SEXERCISE STATS

Energy burn	Energy burn
★★★	★★☆

Muscles used

Triceps
Core
Glutes

Core
Glutes
Quads

Flexibility	Flexibility
★★★	★☆☆

🕐 Keep at it for 5–10 minutes

The longer you go, the more you feel the burn in your triceps

They feel the burn in their quads as they push up and down

You strengthen your glutes as you thrust your hips upward

103

ROCK AND ROLL

Rock to the rhythm of your lovemaking: your moans of pleasure are the melody.

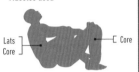
Pulling their partner closer activates their lats

The longer they go, the more their core works

They strengthen their deep core muscles by keeping themselves stable

OFF THE WALL

When you're raring to go and don't want to wait to find a bed, create a seat with your body and have them lunge over your lap.

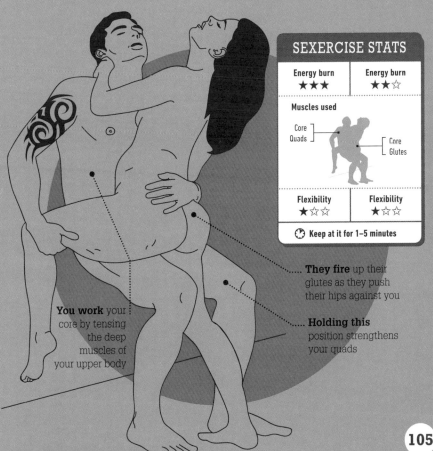

SEXERCISE STATS

Energy burn	Energy burn
★★★	★★☆

Muscles used

Core
Quads

Core
Glutes

Flexibility	Flexibility
★☆☆	★☆☆

🕐 Keep at it for 1–5 minutes

They fire up their glutes as they push their hips against you

Holding this position strengthens your quads

You work your core by tensing the deep muscles of your upper body

HOOKED UP

You hug your partner's legs close to your chest, and they give you a voyeuristic view of their body stretched out before you.

SEXERCISE STATS

Energy burn	Energy burn
★★★	★★★

Muscles used

Deltoids
Arms
Core

Biceps
Glutes
Quads

Flexibility	Flexibility
★★★	★☆☆

🕐 Keep at it for 1–5 minutes

Holding this position strengthens your quads

They work their core by holding themselves up

Holding this position tests their arm strength to the limit

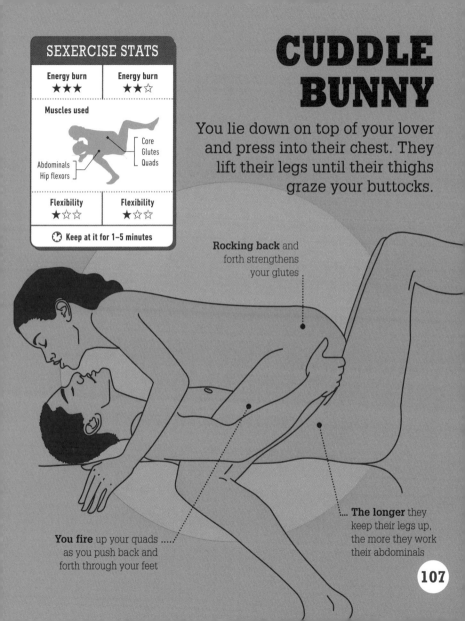

SEXERCISE STATS

Energy burn	Energy burn
★★★	★★☆

Muscles used

Abdominals
Hip flexors

Core
Glutes
Quads

Flexibility	Flexibility
★☆☆	★☆☆

🕐 Keep at it for 1–5 minutes

CUDDLE BUNNY

You lie down on top of your lover and press into their chest. They lift their legs until their thighs graze your buttocks.

Rocking back and forth strengthens your glutes

The longer they keep their legs up, the more they work their abdominals

You fire up your quads as you push back and forth through your feet

AMOROUS ACROBATICS

Lift your legs and challenge your partner to enter. You earn the right to boast about this position when you conquer it.

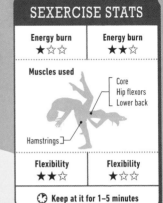
Maintaining this position boosts the strength in your lower back

Their hamstrings get a deep stretch

You fire up your core strength to hold your lower body in this pose

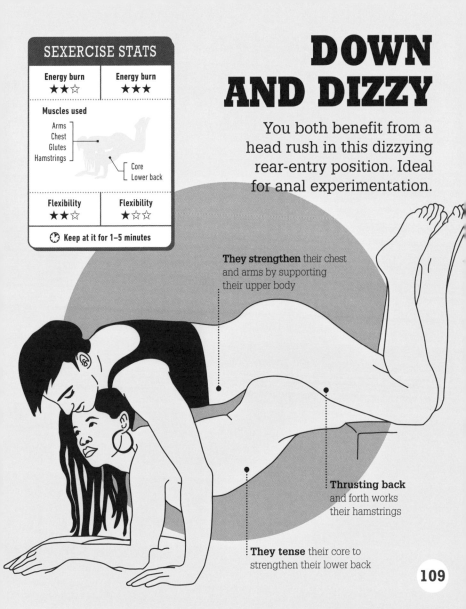

SEXERCISE STATS

Energy burn ★★☆	**Energy burn** ★★★

Muscles used

Arms
Chest
Glutes
Hamstrings

Core
Lower back

Flexibility ★★☆	**Flexibility** ★☆☆

🕐 **Keep at it for 1–5 minutes**

DOWN AND DIZZY

You both benefit from a head rush in this dizzying rear-entry position. Ideal for anal experimentation.

They strengthen their chest and arms by supporting their upper body

Thrusting back and forth works their hamstrings

They tense their core to strengthen their lower back

A TIGHT HOLD

Slow but sensual: you support your lover as they lean back and tighten themselves around you. Take your time finding the perfect fit.

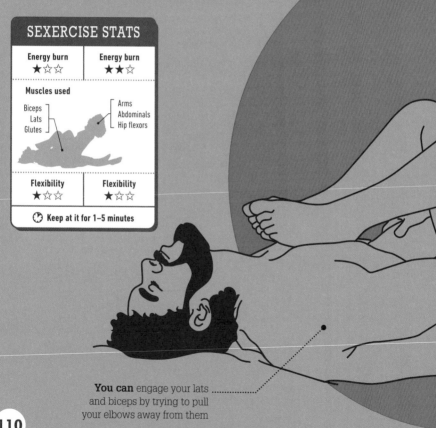

SEXERCISE STATS

Energy burn	Energy burn
★☆☆	★★☆

Muscles used

Biceps
Lats
Glutes

Arms
Abdominals
Hip flexors

Flexibility	Flexibility
★☆☆	★☆☆

🕐 Keep at it for 1–5 minutes

You can engage your lats and biceps by trying to pull your elbows away from them

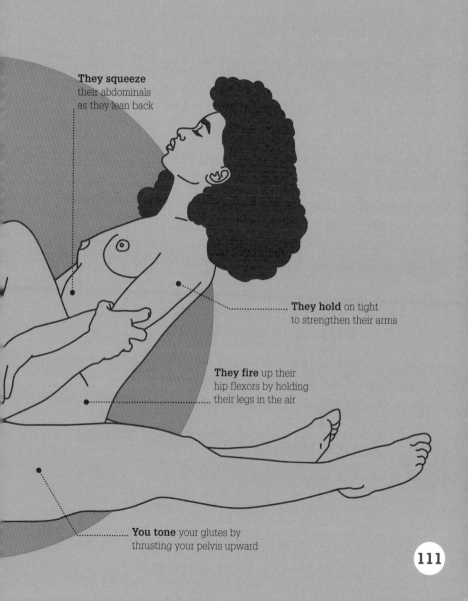

They squeeze their abdominals as they lean back

They hold on tight to strengthen their arms

They fire up their hip flexors by holding their legs in the air

You tone your glutes by thrusting your pelvis upward

111

HEAVENLY STEPS

Your partner plays Cupid in this divine position and pierces you with their love-arrow.

Gripping their waist with your thighs works your adductors

Pushing their hips back and forth strengthens their glutes

You feel the burn in your core muscles

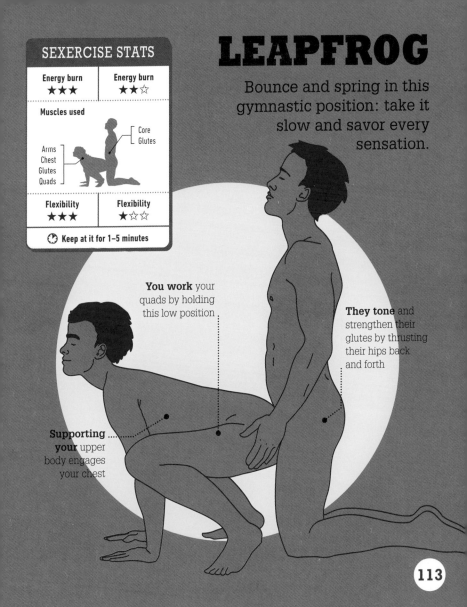

LEAPFROG

Bounce and spring in this gymnastic position: take it slow and savor every sensation.

You work your quads by holding this low position

They tone and strengthen their glutes by thrusting their hips back and forth

Supporting your upper body engages your chest

113

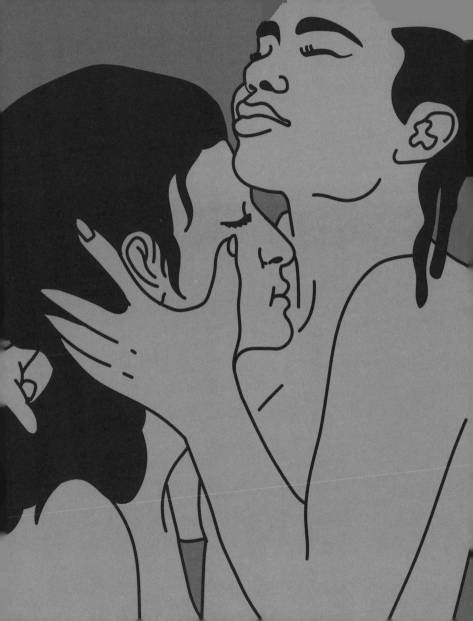

" WHEN THEY GET ON TOP
THEY THEN
SHOW ALL
THEIR LOVE
AND
desire "

THE KAMA SUTRA

STRADDLE UP

Your lover leans back and admires your chest, while you are free to set the pace of passion. They make you melt by caressing your inner thighs.

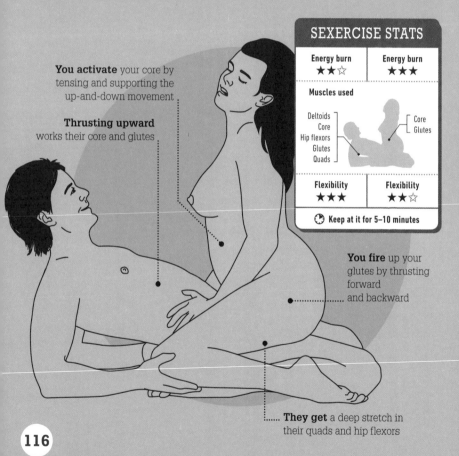

You activate your core by tensing and supporting the up-and-down movement

Thrusting upward works their core and glutes

SEXERCISE STATS

Energy burn	Energy burn
★★☆	★★★

Muscles used

Deltoids
Core
Hip flexors
Glutes
Quads

Core
Glutes

Flexibility	Flexibility
★★★	★★☆

🕐 Keep at it for 5–10 minutes

You fire up your glutes by thrusting forward and backward

They get a deep stretch in their quads and hip flexors

PUSH AND PULL

They tease you by rocking in and out of reach. You can caress their torso and take time to kiss, lick, or nibble their nipples.

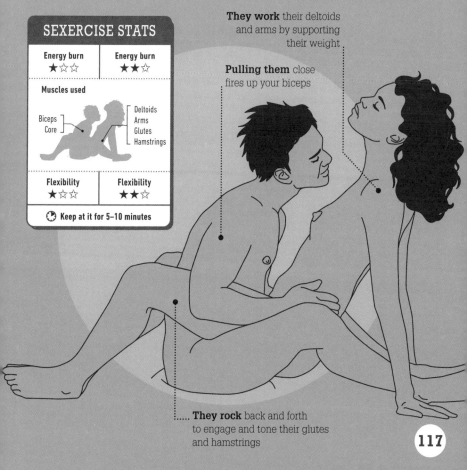

SEXERCISE STATS

Energy burn	Energy burn
★☆☆	★★☆

Muscles used

Biceps
Core

Deltoids
Arms
Glutes
Hamstrings

Flexibility	Flexibility
★☆☆	★★☆

🕐 Keep at it for 5–10 minutes

They work their deltoids and arms by supporting their weight

Pulling them close fires up your biceps

They rock back and forth to engage and tone their glutes and hamstrings

A LOVING BRACE

You caress their thighs and sink between them. They can brace themselves on their forearms to meet your thrusts.

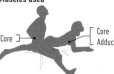
You activate your core around your navel to maintain this position

They fire up their adductors to grip your waist

They rock back and forth through their forearms to work their core

118

LEAN ON ME

Start on top of your lover, then they can take the lead by lifting their knees and leaning you back. They can bounce you gently as you relax and enjoy the ride.

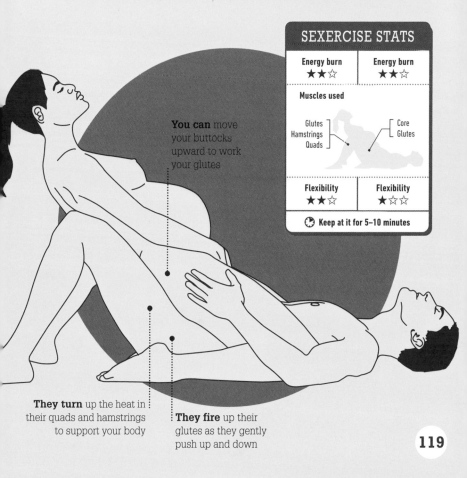

You can move your buttocks upward to work your glutes

SEXERCISE STATS

Energy burn	Energy burn
★★☆	★★☆

Muscles used

Glutes Hamstrings Quads	Core Glutes

Flexibility	Flexibility
★★☆	★☆☆

🕑 **Keep at it for 5–10 minutes**

They turn up the heat in their quads and hamstrings to support your body

They fire up their glutes as they gently push up and down

119

GALLOP TO THE FINISH LINE

Grip your lover's waist hard between your thighs to spur them on. They take a hold of your ankles and lean forward to giddy up.

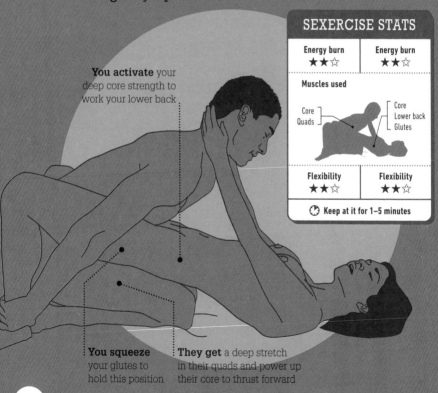

You activate your deep core strength to work your lower back

SEXERCISE STATS

Energy burn	Energy burn
★★☆	★★☆

Muscles used

Core
Quads

Core
Lower back
Glutes

Flexibility	Flexibility
★★☆	★★☆

🕑 Keep at it for 1–5 minutes

You squeeze your glutes to hold this position

They get a deep stretch in their quads and power up their core to thrust forward

HOT HIP HINGE

Lifting one leg makes this rear-entry position super saucy. Use a wall for support so your lover can power it home as hard as you like.

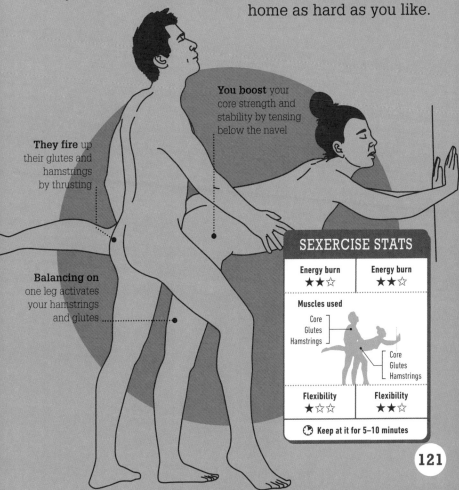

They fire up their glutes and hamstrings by thrusting

You boost your core strength and stability by tensing below the navel

Balancing on one leg activates your hamstrings and glutes

SEXERCISE STATS

Energy burn	Energy burn
★★☆	★★☆

Muscles used

Core
Glutes
Hamstrings

Core
Glutes
Hamstrings

Flexibility	Flexibility
★☆☆	★★☆

🕐 Keep at it for 5–10 minutes

KNEE DEEP

A red-hot position for feverish lovemaking—you can use your knee to rock your lover gently while you both hold on tight and thrust wildly.

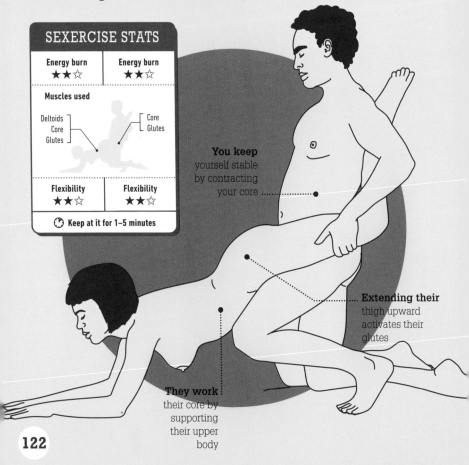

SEXERCISE STATS

Energy burn	Energy burn
★★☆	★★☆

Muscles used

Deltoids
Core
Glutes

Core
Glutes

Flexibility	Flexibility
★★☆	★★☆

🕐 Keep at it for 1–5 minutes

You keep yourself stable by contracting your core

Extending their thigh upward activates their glutes

They work their core by supporting their upper body

SPOONING SWEETHEARTS

Turn your bedtime cuddle into something saucier. You lift your leg and let your lover in from behind.

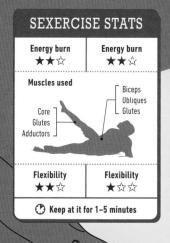

SEXERCISE STATS

Energy burn ★★☆	Energy burn ★★☆

Muscles used

Biceps
Obliques
Glutes

Core
Glutes
Adductors

Flexibility ★★☆	Flexibility ★☆☆

🕑 **Keep at it for 1–5 minutes**

The longer they hold your thigh up, the more they work their biceps

You stretch your adductors by maintaining this position

Thrusting on their side fires up their obliques

JOY RIDE

Your partner fires up their engine and you take them for a spin. When they run out of fuel, switch to an easier position.

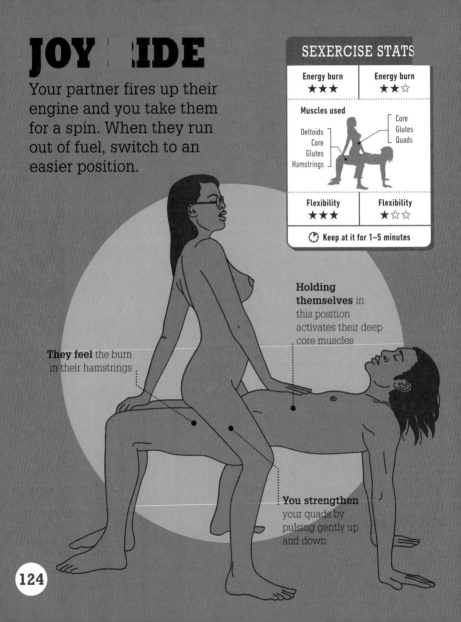

Holding themselves in this position activates their deep core muscles

They feel the burn in their hamstrings

You strengthen your quads by pulsing gently up and down

124

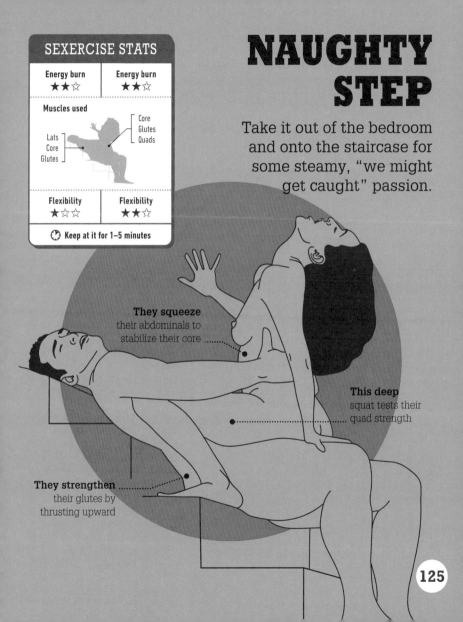

NAUGHTY STEP

Take it out of the bedroom and onto the staircase for some steamy, "we might get caught" passion.

SEXERCISE STATS

Energy burn ★★☆	Energy burn ★★☆

Muscles used

Lats
Core
Glutes

Core
Glutes
Quads

Flexibility ★☆☆	Flexibility ★★☆

🕐 Keep at it for 1–5 minutes

They squeeze their abdominals to stabilize their core

This deep squat tests their quad strength

They strengthen their glutes by thrusting upward

125

G-SPOT GYMNASTICS

What this position lacks in face-to-face intimacy, it more than makes up for in naughtiness. Lose yourselves in your own worlds of sexual bliss.

SEXERCISE STATS

Energy burn	Energy burn
★★☆	★★☆

Muscles used

Abdominals
Core
Glutes
Hip flexors

Deltoids
Chest
Arms
Core
Glutes

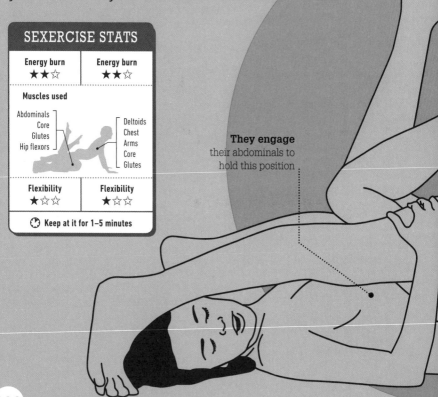

Flexibility	Flexibility
★☆☆	★☆☆

🕐 Keep at it for 1–5 minutes

They engage their abdominals to hold this position

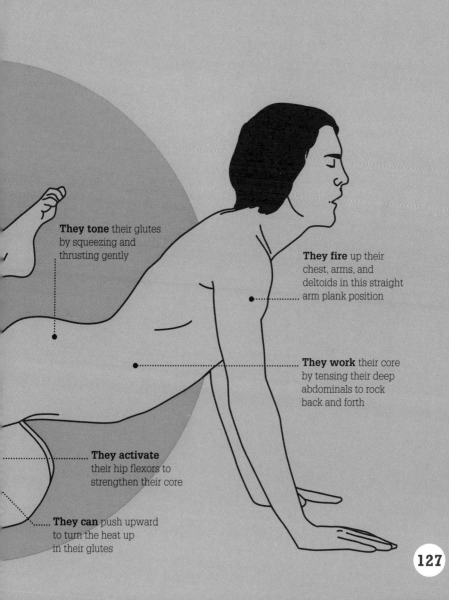

They tone their glutes by squeezing and thrusting gently

They fire up their chest, arms, and deltoids in this straight arm plank position

They work their core by tensing their deep abdominals to rock back and forth

They activate their hip flexors to strengthen their core

They can push upward to turn the heat up in their glutes

127

CROSS-LEGGED CONSUMMATION

This position hits the spot for passionate kisses and sultry skin contact. Luxuriate in your lover's affection.

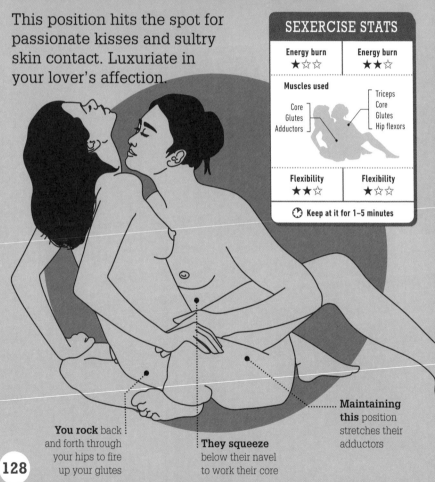

SEXERCISE STATS

Energy burn	Energy burn
★☆☆	★★☆

Muscles used

Core
Glutes
Adductors

Triceps
Core
Glutes
Hip flexors

Flexibility	Flexibility
★★☆	★☆☆

🕐 Keep at it for 1–5 minutes

You rock back and forth through your hips to fire up your glutes

They squeeze below their navel to work their core

Maintaining this position stretches their adductors

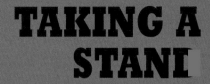

TAKING A STAND

Ideal for fast and feverish loving. Hold your lover tight and let them guide you to their sweet spot.

You thrust your hips back and forth to activate your glutes

They engage their hip flexors by lifting one leg onto a support

Pushing upward through their toes works their calves

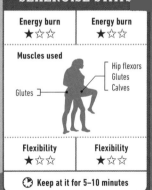

SEXERCISE STATS

Energy burn	Energy burn
★☆☆	★☆☆

Muscles used

Glutes ⅃

Hip flexors
Glutes
Calves

Flexibility	Flexibility
★☆☆	★☆☆

🕐 Keep at it for 5–10 minutes

THE HOT SQUAT

Take control in this steamy squat position. You can choose to keep it tantalizingly slow or to ride your lover fast to the finish line.

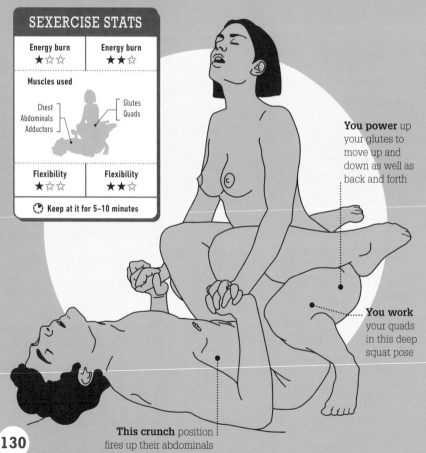

SEXERCISE STATS

Energy burn	Energy burn
★☆☆	★★☆

Muscles used

Chest
Abdominals
Adductors

Glutes
Quads

Flexibility	Flexibility
★☆☆	★★☆

🕐 **Keep at it for 5–10 minutes**

You power up your glutes to move up and down as well as back and forth

You work your quads in this deep squat pose

This crunch position fires up their abdominals

TOUCHING DISTANCE

You can admire their beautiful body from afar. Paying close attention to their erogenous zones while giving plenty of internal stimulation will bring them to an earth-shattering climax.

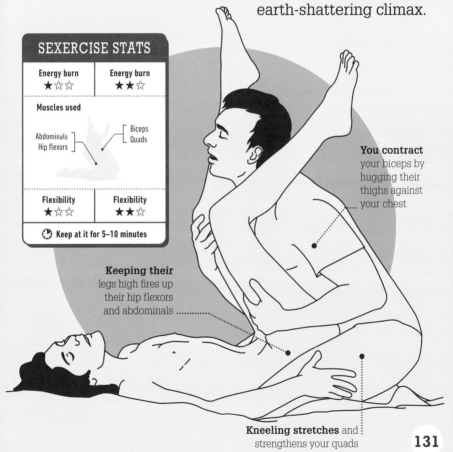

You contract your biceps by hugging their thighs against your chest

Keeping their legs high fires up their hip flexors and abdominals ....

Kneeling stretches and strengthens your quads

131

VOLUPTUOUS V SIT

They clasp hold of you and lean back as far as they dare while you try to rein them in. Pulling them in harder pushes their thighs erotically against your chest.

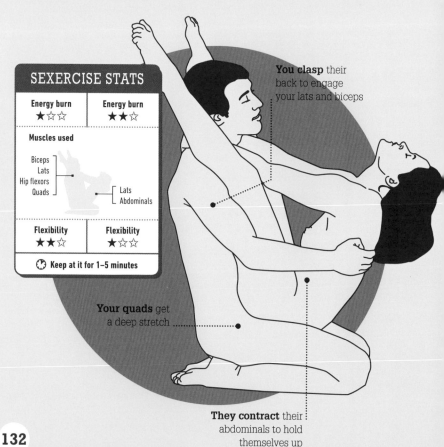

SEXERCISE STATS

Energy burn	Energy burn
★☆☆	★★☆

Muscles used

Biceps
Lats
Hip flexors
Quads

Lats
Abdominals

Flexibility	Flexibility
★★☆	★☆☆

🕑 **Keep at it for 1–5 minutes**

You clasp their back to engage your lats and biceps

Your quads get a deep stretch

They contract their abdominals to hold themselves up

THE THIGH HUMP

You straddle their thigh and rub yourself up and down until they're dying to plunge in deep. The higher you move up their leg, the harder it is for them to resist.

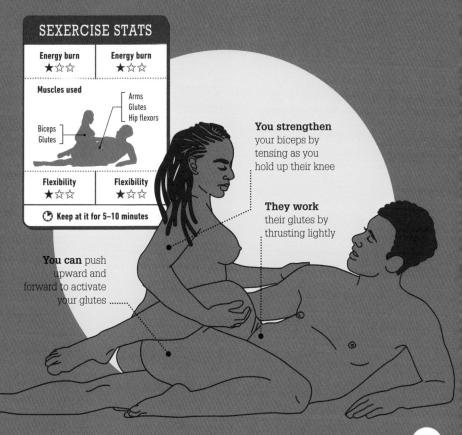

SEXERCISE STATS

Energy burn	Energy burn
★☆☆	★☆☆

Muscles used

Biceps
Glutes

Arms
Glutes
Hip flexors

Flexibility	Flexibility
★☆☆	★☆☆

🕐 **Keep at it for 5–10 minutes**

You strengthen your biceps by tensing as you hold up their knee

They work their glutes by thrusting lightly

You can push upward and forward to activate your glutes

SIX-LEGGED LOVEMAKING

Try this ambitious position when you're feeling playful. Resting your legs on their shoulders locks them in tight while you rock and grind against each other.

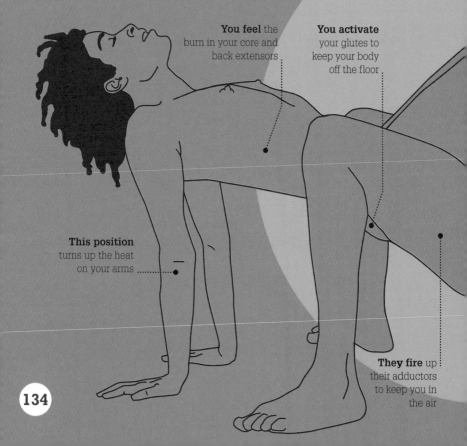

You feel the burn in your core and back extensors

You activate your glutes to keep your body off the floor

This position turns up the heat on your arms

They fire up their adductors to keep you in the air

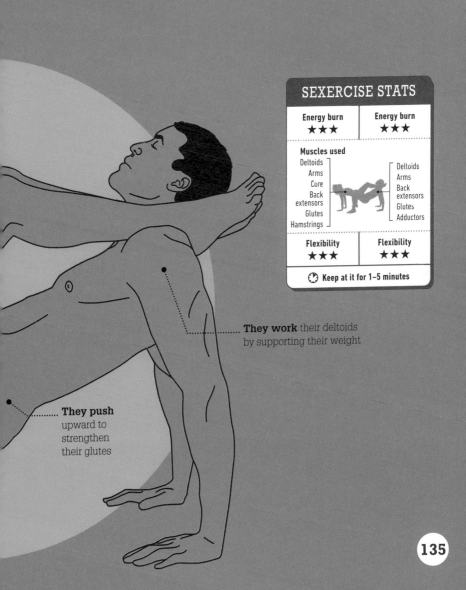

SEXERCISE STATS

Energy burn	Energy burn
★ ★ ★	★ ★ ★

Muscles used

Deltoids
Arms
Core
Back extensors
Glutes
Hamstrings

Deltoids
Arms
Back extensors
Glutes
Adductors

Flexibility	Flexibility
★ ★ ★	★ ★ ★

🕐 Keep at it for 1–5 minutes

They work their deltoids by supporting their weight

They push upward to strengthen their glutes

135

EXOTIC HEADREST

This position is as naughty as it is novel. Your lover raises their legs and you slip underneath.

SEXERCISE STATS

Energy burn	Energy burn
★★☆	★★☆

Muscles used

Core	Abdominals
Glutes	Hip flexors
Quads	Glutes
Hamstrings	

Flexibility	Flexibility
★☆☆	★☆☆

🕐 Keep at it for 1–5 minutes

They feel the burn in their abdominals as they squeeze their hips upward

Keeping contact with their buttocks works your glutes

Thrusting their hips forward fires up their glutes

BUILDING BRIDGES

A true feat of sexual engineering: you support your lover with your bulging biceps, and they get a heady rush.

You thrust forward with your hips to fire up your glutes

SEXERCISE STATS

Energy burn	Energy burn
★★☆	★★★

Muscles used

Biceps
Core
Glutes

Deltoids
Traps
Hip flexors
Calves

Flexibility	Flexibility
★☆☆	★★★

🕐 **Keep at it for 1–5 minutes**

They strengthen their traps as they lean backward

Standing on tiptoe works their calves

137

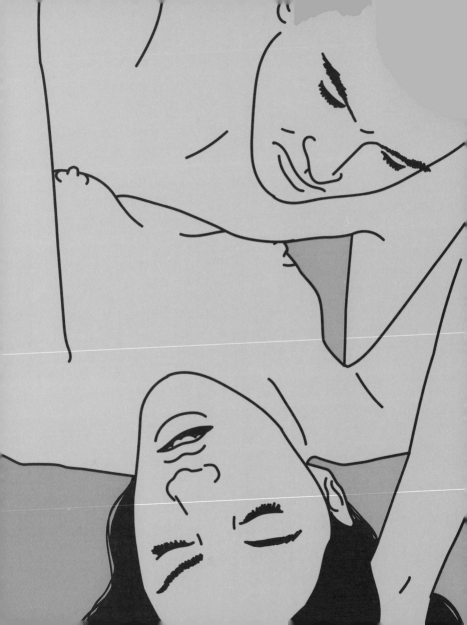

" **THE LIMBS OF BOTH** *touching,* *entangled* **WITH THE** **CORRESPONDING** **PARTS OF THE OTHER** "

THE ANANGA RANGA

RIDGE OF SI⬛⬛S

Take this opportunity to watch penetration from an unusual angle, or enjoy focusing solely on your own pleasure.

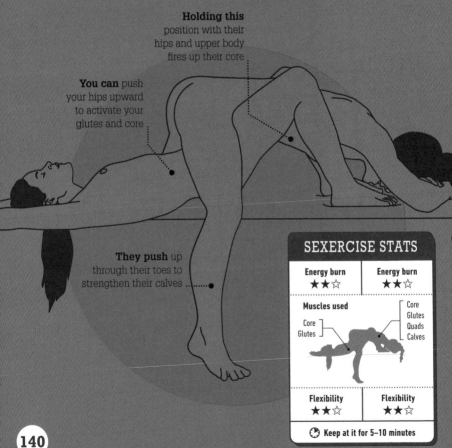

Holding this position with their hips and upper body fires up their core

You can push your hips upward to activate your glutes and core

They push up through their toes to strengthen their calves

SEXERCISE STATS

Energy burn ★★☆	Energy burn ★★☆
Muscles used Core Glutes	Core Glutes Quads Calves
Flexibility ★★☆	Flexibility ★★☆

🕑 Keep at it for 5–10 minutes

THE BALL BOUNCER

Your partner grasps hold of your hands and bobs up and down on you. You can squeeze them between your thighs for some sexy skin-on-skin friction.

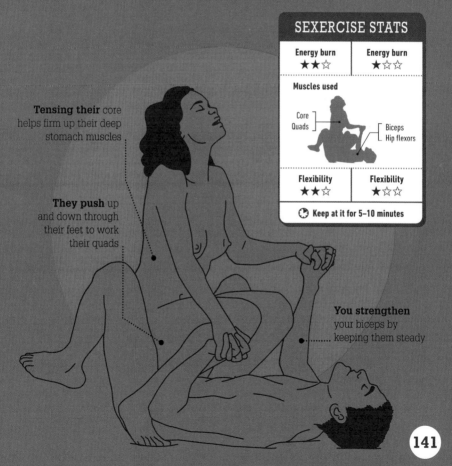

Tensing their core helps firm up their deep stomach muscles

They push up and down through their feet to work their quads

You strengthen your biceps by keeping them steady

SEXERCISE STATS

Energy burn ★★☆	Energy burn ★☆☆
Muscles used	
Core Quads	Biceps Hip flexors
Flexibility ★★☆	Flexibility ★☆☆

🕐 Keep at it for 5–10 minutes

PRESS THE FLESH

You lean back and bare your chest. Pushing your knees together makes them feel even tighter inside you.

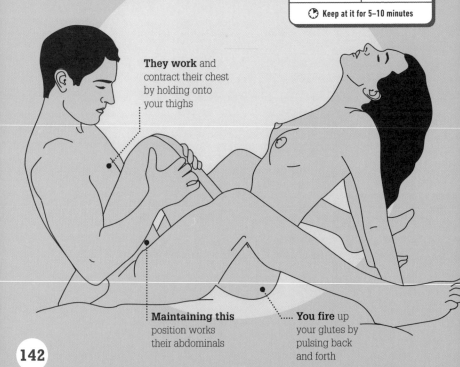

They work and contract their chest by holding onto your thighs

Maintaining this position works their abdominals

You fire up your glutes by pulsing back and forth

142

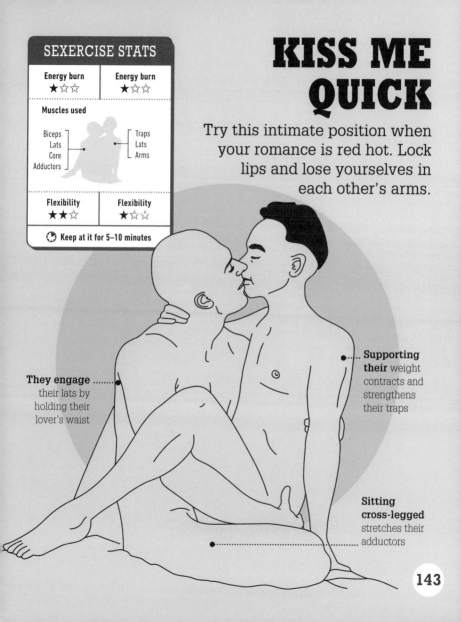

SEXERCISE STATS

Energy burn	Energy burn
★☆☆	★☆☆

Muscles used

Biceps	Traps
Lats	Lats
Core	Arms
Adductors	

Flexibility	Flexibility
★★☆	★☆☆

🕑 Keep at it for 5–10 minutes

KISS ME QUICK

Try this intimate position when your romance is red hot. Lock lips and lose yourselves in each other's arms.

Supporting their weight contracts and strengthens their traps

They engage their lats by holding their lover's waist

Sitting cross-legged stretches their adductors

143

SENSUAL SIT-UP

Stare lovingly at each other from a tantalizing distance. Your lover grips your upper body between their legs and leans back so you can enjoy an erotic view.

SEXERCISE STATS

Energy burn	Energy burn
★★☆	★★★

Muscles used

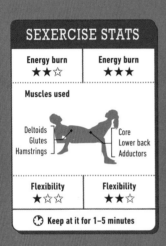

Deltoids
Glutes
Hamstrings

Core
Lower back
Adductors

Flexibility	Flexibility
★☆☆	★★☆

🕐 Keep at it for 1–5 minutes

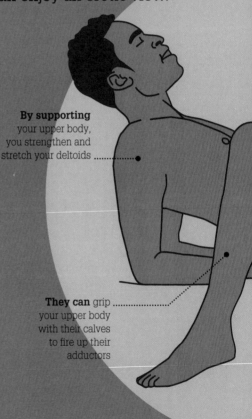

By supporting your upper body, you strengthen and stretch your deltoids ....•

They can grip .... your upper body with their calves to fire up their adductors

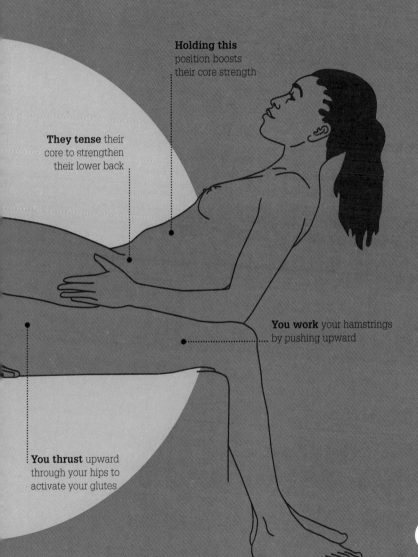

Holding this position boosts their core strength

They tense their core to strengthen their lower back

You work your hamstrings by pushing upward

You thrust upward through your hips to activate your glutes

145

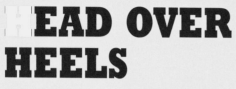

HEAD OVER HEELS

Enjoy the erotic drama of this impressive pose. You can push yourself off the wall to rock back and forth for more stimulation.

SEXERCISE STATS

Energy burn	Energy burn
★★☆	★★☆

Muscles used

Deltoids ⎤	⎡ Arms
Arms	Lats
Core	Glutes
Hamstrings ⎦	Quads
	⎣ Hamstrings

Flexibility	Flexibility
★★☆	★☆☆

🕒 Keep at it for 1–5 minutes

They hold your thighs to strengthen their lats and arms

Supporting your upper body weight activates your deltoids and arms

They thrust from behind to work their glutes

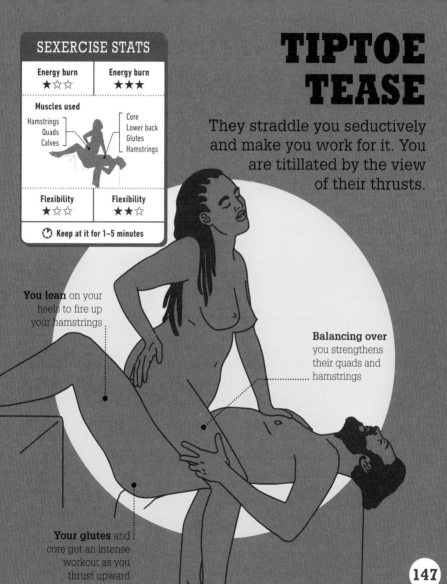

TIPTOE TEASE

They straddle you seductively and make you work for it. You are titillated by the view of their thrusts.

SEXERCISE STATS

Energy burn ★☆☆	Energy burn ★★★

Muscles used

Hamstrings
Quads
Calves

Core
Lower back
Glutes
Hamstrings

Flexibility ★☆☆	Flexibility ★★☆

🕐 Keep at it for 1–5 minutes

You lean on your heels to fire up your hamstrings

Balancing over you strengthens their quads and hamstrings

Your glutes and core get an intense workout as you thrust upward

147

BUNNY HO

A compact variation of the wheelbarrow: you slide onto your partner and they lift you by the ankles, then you both go at it like rabbits.

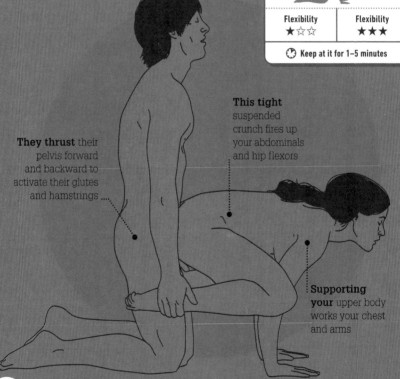

This tight suspended crunch fires up your abdominals and hip flexors

They thrust their pelvis forward and backward to activate their glutes and hamstrings

Supporting your upper body works your chest and arms

148

TEASE ON TOP

Your lover bounces on top to keep you just on the edge until you're both ready to explode. Squeeze each other's hands as the tension mounts.

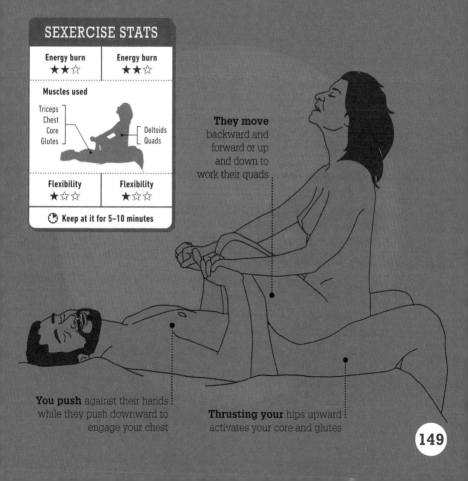

SEXERCISE STATS

Energy burn ★★☆	Energy burn ★★☆

Muscles used

Triceps
Chest
Core
Glutes

Deltoids
Quads

Flexibility ★☆☆	Flexibility ★☆☆

🕑 Keep at it for 5–10 minutes

They move backward and forward or up and down to work their quads

You push against their hands while they push downward to engage your chest

Thrusting your hips upward activates your core and glutes

149

SEXY STRONGHOLD

Climb up your lover and clasp hold tightly. Don't let each other go until your desires are fully satiated.

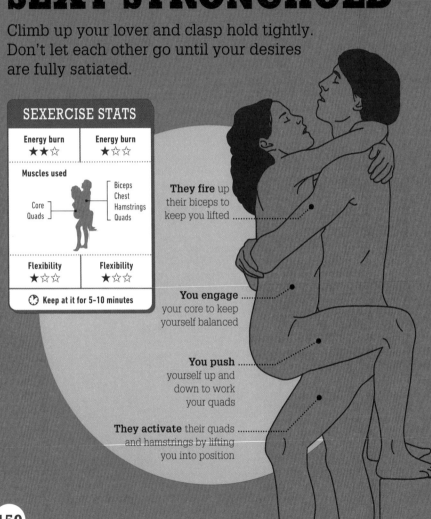

SEXERCISE STATS

Energy burn	Energy burn
★★☆	★☆☆

Muscles used

Core
Quads

Biceps
Chest
Hamstrings
Quads

Flexibility	Flexibility
★☆☆	★☆☆

🕐 Keep at it for 5–10 minutes

They fire up their biceps to keep you lifted

You engage your core to keep yourself balanced

You push yourself up and down to work your quads

They activate their quads and hamstrings by lifting you into position

RACE CAR DRIVER

You are the driver's seat, and they push all your pedals. They start slowly, then accelerate. Go full speed until you both cross the finish line.

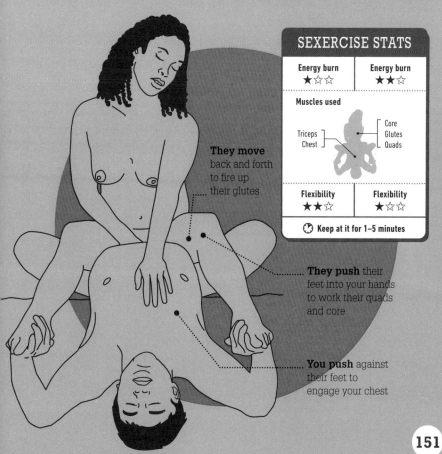

SEXERCISE STATS

Energy burn	Energy burn
★☆☆	★★☆

Muscles used

Triceps
Chest

Core
Glutes
Quads

Flexibility	Flexibility
★★☆	★☆☆

🕐 **Keep at it for 1–5 minutes**

They move back and forth to fire up their glutes

They push their feet into your hands to work their quads and core

You push against their feet to engage your chest

BALANCE OF BLISS

Your lover forms a stiff bridge with their body and lets you test out the suspension. They can massage your buttocks or lie back and enjoy being taken by you.

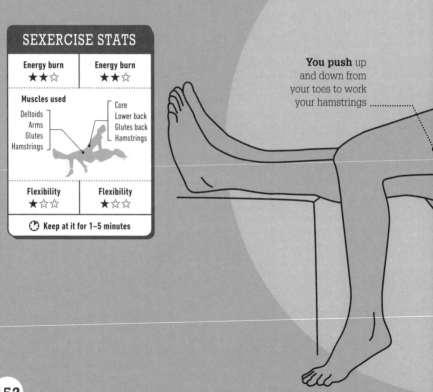

SEXERCISE STATS

Energy burn	Energy burn
★★☆	★★☆

Muscles used

Deltoids
Arms
Glutes
Hamstrings

Core
Lower back
Glutes back
Hamstrings

Flexibility	Flexibility
★☆☆	★☆☆

🕐 Keep at it for 1–5 minutes

You push up and down from your toes to work your hamstrings

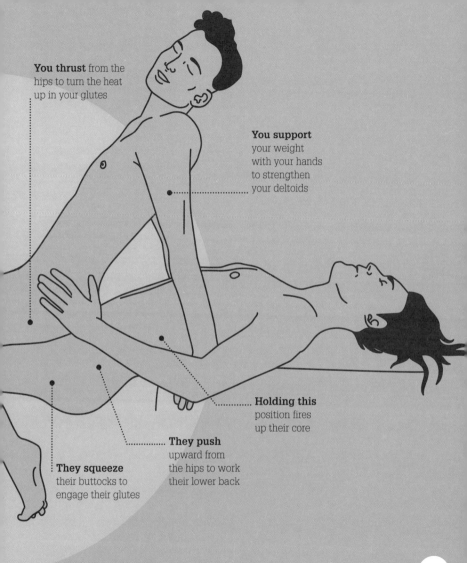

You thrust from the hips to turn the heat up in your glutes

You support your weight with your hands to strengthen your deltoids

Holding this position fires up their core

They push upward from the hips to work their lower back

They squeeze their buttocks to engage their glutes

153

TEASE TO PLEASE

Get adventurous and see if you can make it fit. Only the very tip of you will make an entrance, so it's ideal for exotic presex titillation.

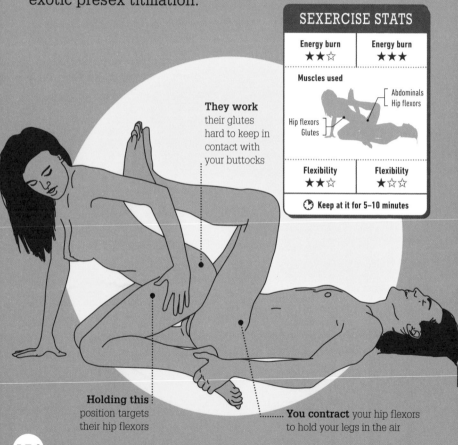

SEXERCISE STATS

Energy burn	Energy burn
★★☆	★★★

Muscles used

Abdominals
Hip flexors

Hip flexors
Glutes

Flexibility	Flexibility
★★☆	★☆☆

⏱ **Keep at it for 5–10 minutes**

They work their glutes hard to keep in contact with your buttocks

Holding this position targets their hip flexors

You contract your hip flexors to hold your legs in the air

POWER PLAY

Fire up the sexual tension with this dramatic position: you push against their chest with your feet while they return the force with the power of their thrusts.

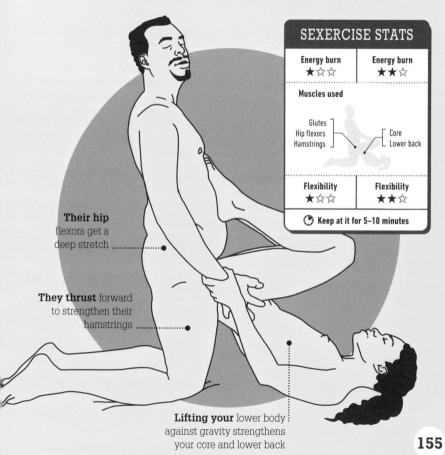

SEXERCISE STATS

Energy burn	Energy burn
★☆☆	★★☆

Muscles used

Glutes
Hip flexors
Hamstrings

Core
Lower back

Flexibility	Flexibility
★☆☆	★★☆

🕐 Keep at it for 5–10 minutes

Their hip flexors get a deep stretch

They thrust forward to strengthen their hamstrings

Lifting your lower body against gravity strengthens your core and lower back

HOLD ME CLOSE

They sit between your legs and shimmy as close as they can. Perfect for languorous kisses.

Moving their hips back and forth engages their glutes

You fire up your hip flexors by sitting in this position and pulsing back and forth

They work their hip flexors in this pose

156

DON'T LET GO

A provocatively taut position: hold onto each other's wrists tightly, then heat it up by leaning apart.

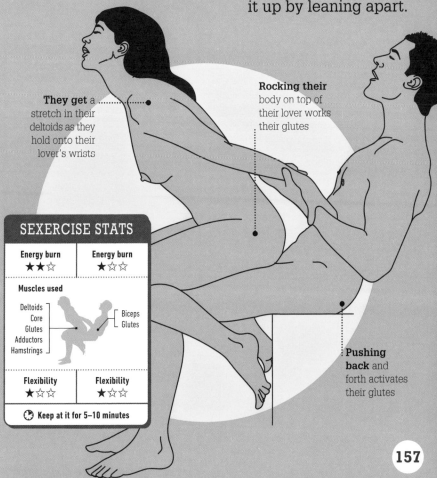

They get a stretch in their deltoids as they hold onto their lover's wrists

Rocking their body on top of their lover works their glutes

Pushing back and forth activates their glutes

SEXERCISE STATS

Energy burn	Energy burn
★★☆	★☆☆

Muscles used

Deltoids
Core
Glutes
Adductors
Hamstrings

Biceps
Glutes

Flexibility	Flexibility
★☆☆	★☆☆

🕐 Keep at it for 5–10 minutes

157

TORRID TEASE

Lean back and succumb to your lover's seduction. You can stroke the back of their thighs to make them tremble with delight.

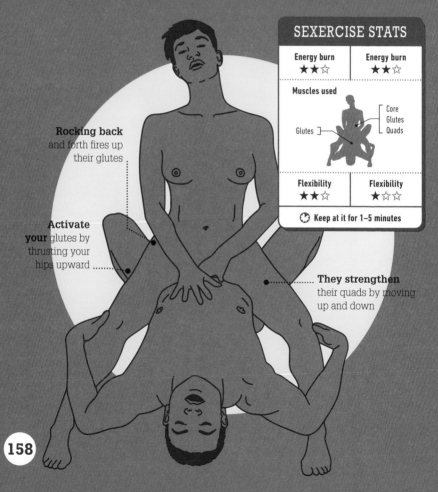

Rocking back and forth fires up their glutes

Activate your glutes by thrusting your hips upward

They strengthen their quads by moving up and down

SEXERCISE STATS

Energy burn	Energy burn
★★☆	★★☆

Muscles used

Glutes]

[Core
Glutes
Quads

Flexibility	Flexibility
★★☆	★☆☆

🕐 Keep at it for 1–5 minutes

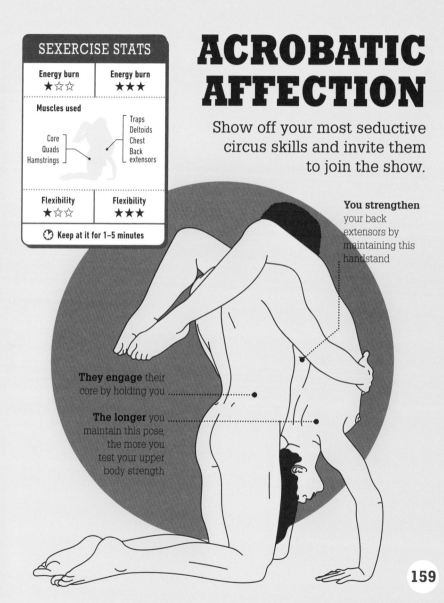

SEXERCISE STATS

Energy burn	Energy burn
★☆☆	★★★

Muscles used

Core
Quads
Hamstrings

Traps
Deltoids
Chest
Back
extensors

Flexibility	Flexibility
★☆☆	★★★

🕑 Keep at it for 1–5 minutes

ACROBATIC AFFECTION

Show off your most seductive circus skills and invite them to join the show.

You strengthen your back extensors by maintaining this handstand

They engage their core by holding you

The longer you maintain this pose, the more you test your upper body strength

159

CLUTCH TO CLIMAX

Your love cranks up the kinkiness by grabbing your legs as they bounce up and down. If you're peaking too quickly, take hold of their buttocks to slow them down.

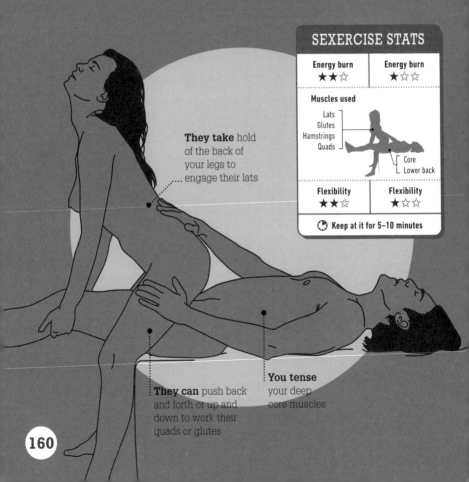

They take hold of the back of your legs to engage their lats

SEXERCISE STATS

Energy burn ★★☆	Energy burn ★☆☆
Muscles used	
Lats Glutes Hamstrings Quads — Core Lower back	
Flexibility ★★☆	Flexibility ★☆☆
🕐 Keep at it for 5–10 minutes	

They can push back and forth or up and down to work their quads or glutes

You tense your deep core muscles

SEXUAL FLEX LEG

Show off your suppleness by raising your leg, then invite them in to explore the unusual sensations of side-entry sex.

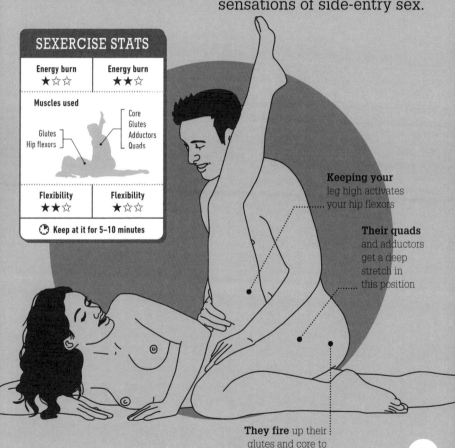

SEXERCISE STATS

Energy burn	Energy burn
★☆☆	★★☆

Muscles used

Glutes
Hip flexors

Core
Glutes
Adductors
Quads

Flexibility	Flexibility
★★☆	★☆☆

🕐 **Keep at it for 5–10 minutes**

Keeping your leg high activates your hip flexors

Their quads and adductors get a deep stretch in this position

They fire up their glutes and core to thrust forward

161

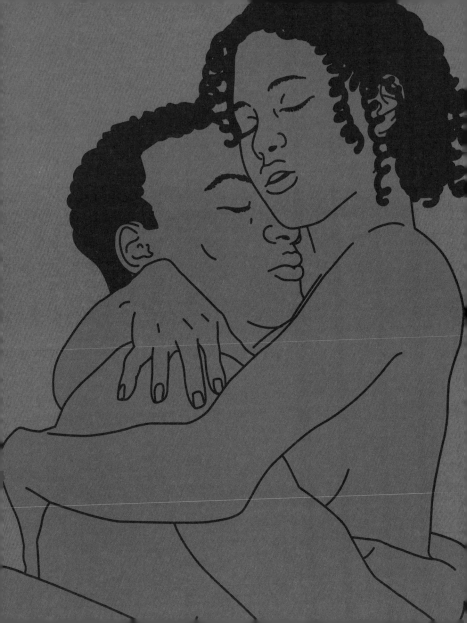

"*Their smiles* BROKEN BY HARD BREATHINGS, THEY SHOULD PRESS AGAINST THEIR *lover's* BOSOM"

THE KAMA SUTRA

COLD SHOULDER

You're each in separate spheres of delight, so let your imagination roam free. You take the lead, but your partner's hands can guide you.

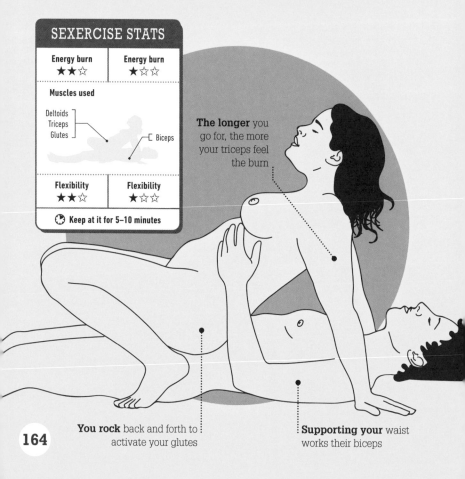

SEXERCISE STATS

Energy burn	Energy burn
★★☆	★☆☆

Muscles used

Deltoids
Triceps
Glutes

Biceps

Flexibility	Flexibility
★★☆	★☆☆

🕑 Keep at it for 5–10 minutes

The longer you go for, the more your triceps feel the burn

You rock back and forth to activate your glutes

Supporting your waist works their biceps

SEDUCTIVE SEAT

The touch of your lover's legs against your body
gets you both going. Take the opportunity
to put your hands to good use.

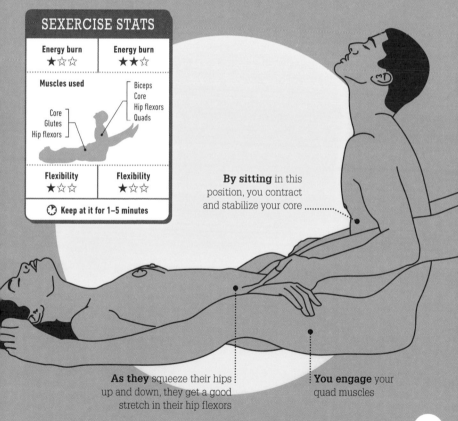

SEXERCISE STATS

Energy burn	Energy burn
★☆☆	★★☆

Muscles used

Core
Glutes
Hip flexors

Biceps
Core
Hip flexors
Quads

Flexibility	Flexibility
★☆☆	★☆☆

🕐 **Keep at it for 1–5 minutes**

By sitting in this
position, you contract
and stabilize your core

As they squeeze their hips
up and down, they get a good
stretch in their hip flexors

You engage your
quad muscles

LEG-LOCKED

Entwine yourselves in each other's limbs and rock back and forth with the tide of your passion.

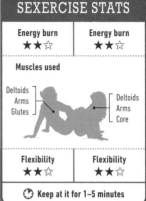

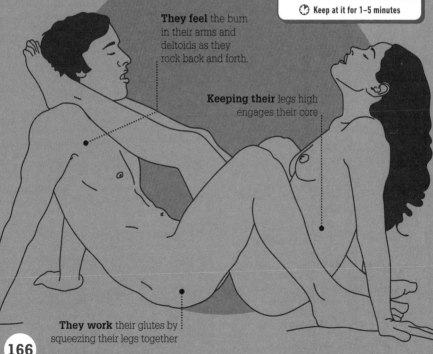

They feel the burn in their arms and deltoids as they rock back and forth.

Keeping their legs high engages their core

They work their glutes by squeezing their legs together

CLIFF-BANGER

Play around on the precipice of pleasure until you both topple over the edge. Your lover gets a handful of your hot buttocks, and you enjoy a dizzying head rush.

The longer they hold your buttocks, the more their triceps feel the burn

They fire up their glutes as they thrust

Maintaining this position works their core and lower back

You engage your chest and deltoids to keep yourself steady

Supporting your upper body strengthens your arms

SEXERCISE STATS

Energy burn ★★☆	Energy burn ★★★
Muscles used	
Deltoids Arms Chest	Triceps Core Lower back Glutes
Flexibility ★☆☆	Flexibility ★★☆

🕐 Keep at it for 1–5 minutes

BOTTOMS UP

Explore the exotic angle of penetration in this hot rear-entry position. Your partner can grab hold of your buttocks and move you into the right spot.

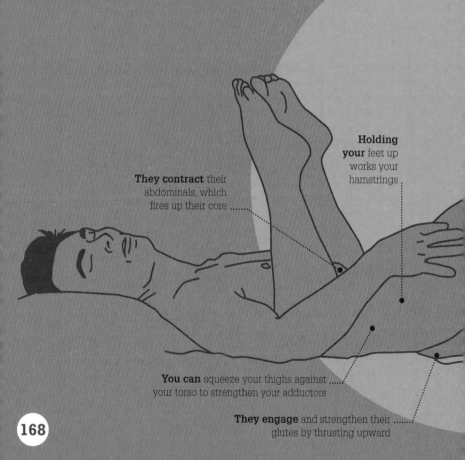

Holding your feet up works your hamstrings

They contract their abdominals, which fires up their core

You can squeeze your thighs against your torso to strengthen your adductors

They engage and strengthen their glutes by thrusting upward

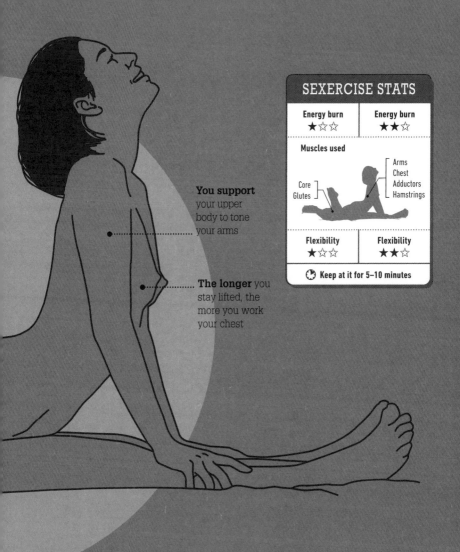

You support your upper body to tone your arms

The longer you stay lifted, the more you work your chest

SEXERCISE STATS

Energy burn	Energy burn
★☆☆	★★☆

Muscles used

Core
Glutes

Arms
Chest
Adductors
Hamstrings

Flexibility	Flexibility
★☆☆	★★☆

🕐 Keep at it for 5–10 minutes

PLEASURE-ME TREE POSE

You both lift one leg, then hold your balance as the sexual energy builds to bliss. Guide your lover to take your pleasure into their own hands.

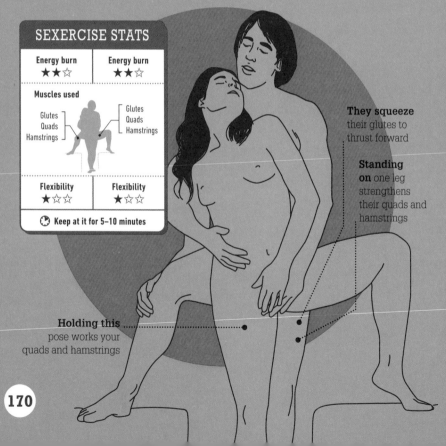

SEXERCISE STATS

Energy burn	Energy burn
★★☆	★★☆

Muscles used

Glutes
Quads
Hamstrings

Glutes
Quads
Hamstrings

Flexibility	Flexibility
★☆☆	★☆☆

🌐 Keep at it for 5–10 minutes

They squeeze their glutes to thrust forward

Standing on one leg strengthens their quads and hamstrings

Holding this pose works your quads and hamstrings

STEAMY STOMACH CRUNCH

Clasp your lover's shoulders as they lean over and grasp your ankles. Then you can both rock yourselves to a sizzling climax.

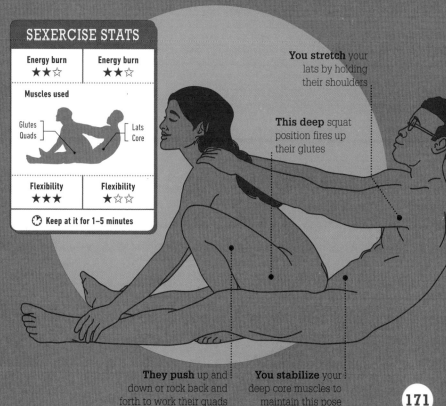

SEXERCISE STATS

Energy burn	Energy burn
★★☆	★★☆

Muscles used

Glutes
Quads — Lats
Core

Flexibility	Flexibility
★★★	★☆☆

🕐 **Keep at it for 1–5 minutes**

You stretch your lats by holding their shoulders

This deep squat position fires up their glutes

They push up and down or rock back and forth to work their quads

You stabilize your deep core muscles to maintain this pose

TUG OF WAR

When the tension between you is at its peak, try battling it out in the bedroom. Clasp hold, lean back, and do your worst.

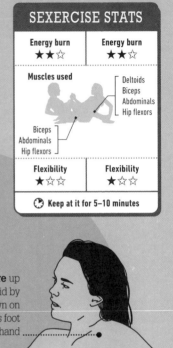
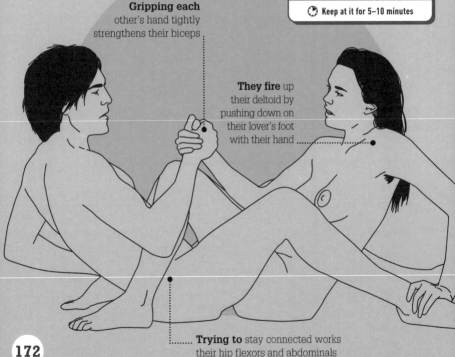

Gripping each other's hand tightly strengthens their biceps

They fire up their deltoid by pushing down on their lover's foot with their hand

Trying to stay connected works their hip flexors and abdominals

172

BLISSFUL BEND

Bend over and let your partner sidle up behind you for some thigh-on-thigh contact. Try pushing your legs against each other for even more erotic friction.

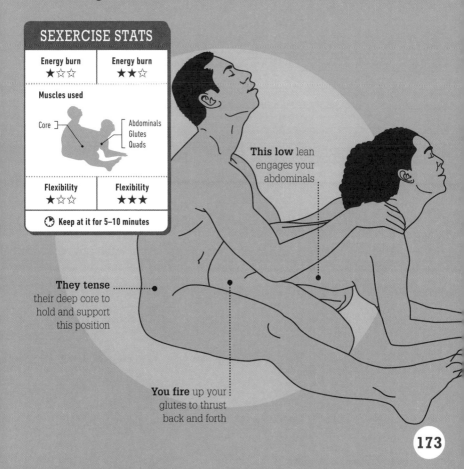

SEXERCISE STATS

Energy burn	Energy burn
★☆☆	★★☆

Muscles used

Core —

Abdominals
Glutes
Quads

Flexibility	Flexibility
★☆☆	★★★

🕑 **Keep at it for 5–10 minutes**

This low lean engages your abdominals

They tense their deep core to hold and support this position

You fire up your glutes to thrust back and forth

LEAN QUEEN

Take a dominating seat on their throne and make them grovel at your feet. They try to overthrow you with the power of their thrusts.

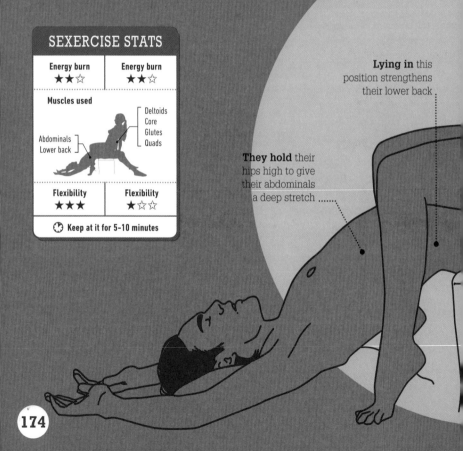

SEXERCISE STATS

Energy burn	Energy burn
★★☆	★★☆

Muscles used

Deltoids
Core
Glutes
Quads

Abdominals
Lower back

Flexibility	Flexibility
★★★	★☆☆

🕐 **Keep at it for 5-10 minutes**

Lying in this position strengthens their lower back

They hold their hips high to give their abdominals a deep stretch

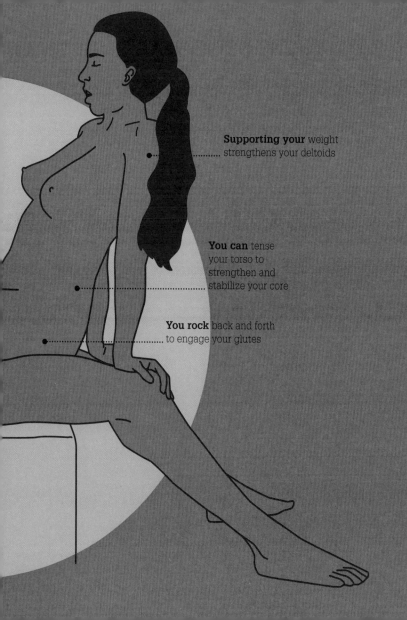

Supporting your weight
.... strengthens your deltoids

You can tense
your torso to
strengthen and
stabilize your core

You rock back and forth
.... to engage your glutes

175

LOVERS' LUNGE

Press your bodies firmly into each other in this saucy standing pose. If penetration proves too tricky, you can slide up and down their thigh for some fiery foreplay.

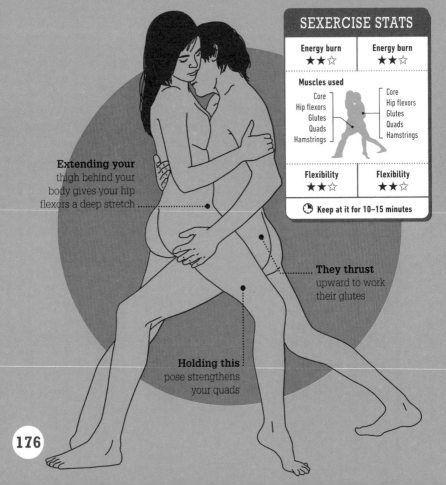

SEXERCISE STATS

Energy burn	Energy burn
★★☆	★★☆

Muscles used

Core	Core
Hip flexors	Hip flexors
Glutes	Glutes
Quads	Quads
Hamstrings	Hamstrings

Flexibility	Flexibility
★★☆	★★☆

🕒 **Keep at it for 10–15 minutes**

Extending your thigh behind your body gives your hip flexors a deep stretch

They thrust upward to work their glutes

Holding this pose strengthens your quads

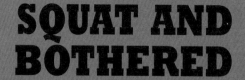

SQUAT AND BOTHERED

Get down and dirty in this deep squat. Hook their ankle over your thigh and keep going until you both feel the heat.

SEXERCISE STATS

Energy burn	Energy burn
★★☆	★☆☆

Muscles used

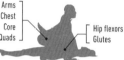

Arms
Chest
Core
Quads

Hip flexors
Glutes

Flexibility	Flexibility
★★☆	★☆☆

🕐 Keep at it for 1–5 minutes

Supporting your weight works your arms and chest

This deep squat fires up your quads

They rest their leg on your thigh to engage their hip flexors

177

BUCK UP

Cross your ankles behind your lover and draw them close. They make you bounce with the power of their thrusts.

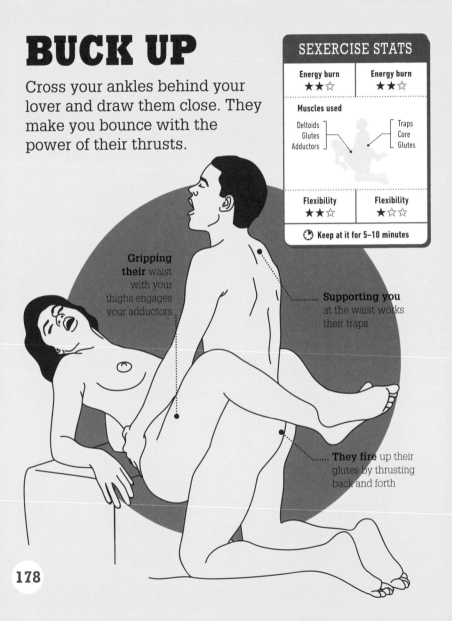

SEXERCISE STATS

Energy burn	Energy burn
★★☆	★★☆

Muscles used

Deltoids
Glutes
Adductors

Traps
Core
Glutes

Flexibility	Flexibility
★★☆	★☆☆

🕐 Keep at it for 5–10 minutes

Gripping their waist with your thighs engages your adductors

Supporting you at the waist works their traps

They fire up their glutes by thrusting back and forth

KOALA CUDDLES

A tender pose to make you both feel warm and fuzzy: lock your partner in, then kiss their neck lovingly.

SEXERCISE STATS

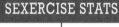

Energy burn	Energy burn
★☆☆	★☆☆

Muscles used

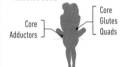

Core
Adductors

Core
Glutes
Quads

Flexibility	Flexibility
★★☆	★☆☆

⏱ Keep at it for 1–5 minutes

Pulsing up and down activates their quads

You stretch your adductors by maintaining this pose

They thrust their hips back and forth to work their glutes

179

CUNNILINGUS CONTORTIONIST

Swing your feet over your head to create a provocative shape with your body. Grabbing hold of your lover's thighs turns up the erotic action.

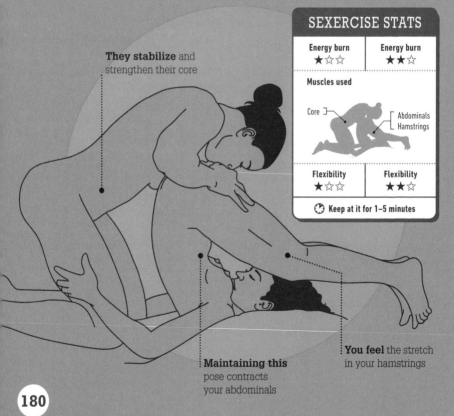

They stabilize and strengthen their core

SEXERCISE STATS

Energy burn	Energy burn
★☆☆	★★☆

Muscles used

Core

Abdominals
Hamstrings

Flexibility	Flexibility
★☆☆	★★☆

🕐 Keep at it for 1–5 minutes

Maintaining this pose contracts your abdominals

You feel the stretch in your hamstrings

Geometry gets juicy: you
lie back on their legs and
they pull your knees
into their chest.

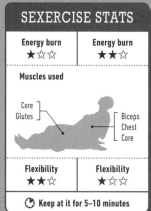

SEXERCISE STATS

Energy burn ★☆☆	Energy burn ★★☆

Muscles used

Core
Glutes

Biceps
Chest
Core

Flexibility ★★☆	Flexibility ★☆☆

🕑 **Keep at it for 5–10 minutes**

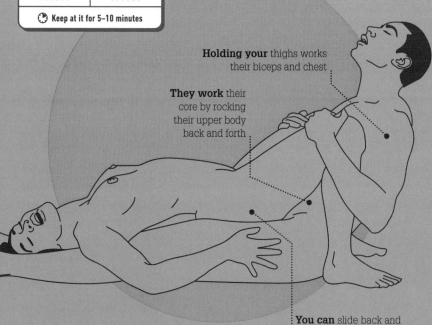

Holding your thighs works
their biceps and chest

They work their
core by rocking
their upper body
back and forth

You can slide back and
forth to tone your glutes

TREASURE MY CHEST

Straddle one of their legs while pressing the other toward their chest. They can stroke your nipples as you lean closer, giving you extra jolts of desire.

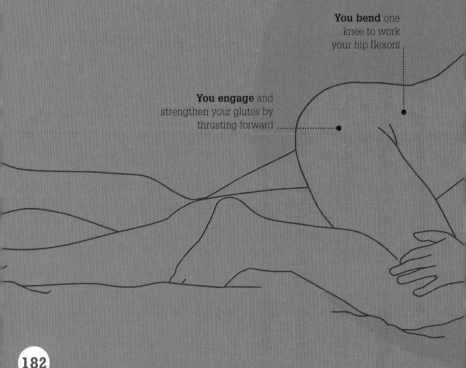

You bend one knee to work your hip flexors

You engage and strengthen your glutes by thrusting forward

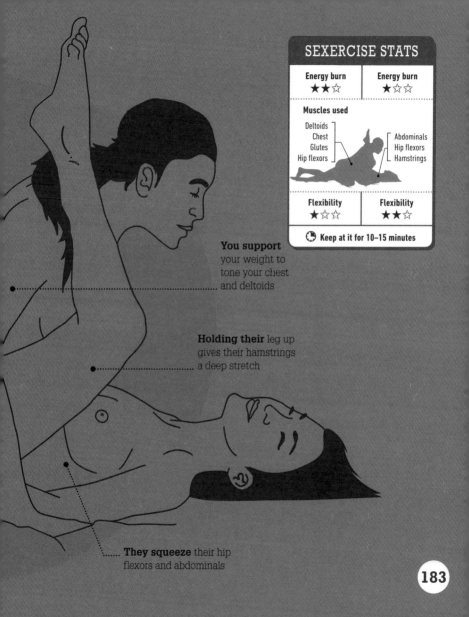

SEXERCISE STATS

Energy burn ★★☆	Energy burn ★☆☆
Muscles used	
Deltoids Chest Glutes Hip flexors	Abdominals Hip flexors Hamstrings
Flexibility ★☆☆	Flexibility ★★☆
🕐 Keep at it for 10–15 minutes	

You support your weight to tone your chest and deltoids

Holding their leg up gives their hamstrings a deep stretch

They squeeze their hip flexors and abdominals

183

DEEPER LOVE

To reach heart-stopping depths,
bring your knees close to your
chest. Supporting your lower back
will help you go the distance.

Supporting their upper body works their chest

They thrust deeply with their hips to activate their glutes

You feel the burn in your hip flexors and abdominals

STRETCH YOUR IMAGINATION

Their legs are the star of the show: they hold them up and you push against them with your chest.

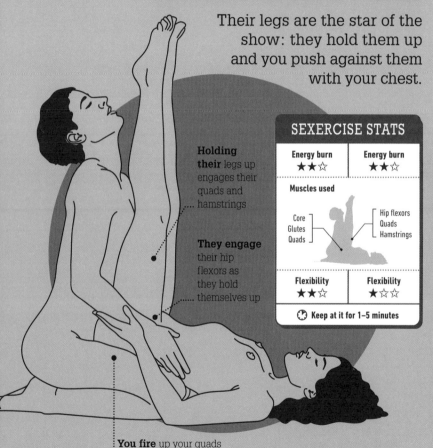

Holding their legs up engages their quads and hamstrings

They engage their hip flexors as they hold themselves up

You fire up your quads as you thrust upward with your hips

SEXERCISE STATS

Energy burn	Energy burn
★★☆	★★☆

Muscles used

Core
Glutes
Quads

Hip flexors
Quads
Hamstrings

Flexibility	Flexibility
★★☆	★☆☆

🕐 **Keep at it for 1–5 minutes**

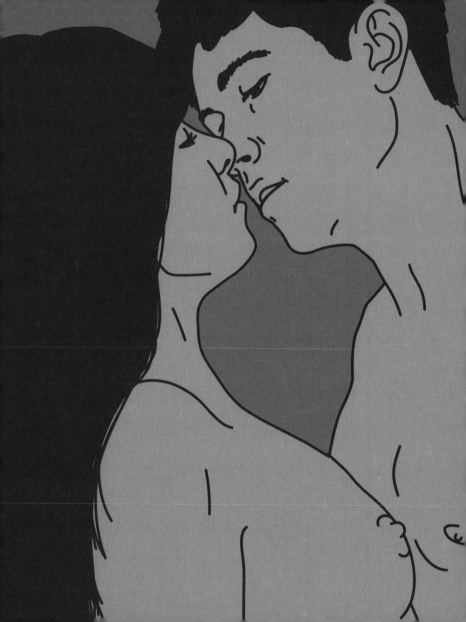

"Excite them

WITH KISSES,
BY NIBBLING AND SUCKING
THEIR LIPS,
BY CARESSING THEIR NECK
AND CHEEKS"

THE PERFUMED GARDEN

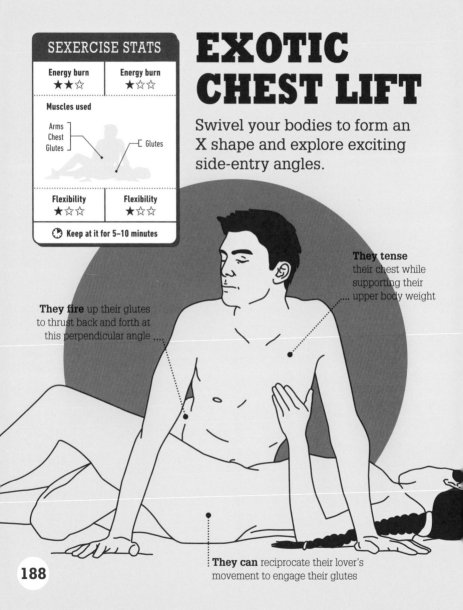

| Energy burn | Energy burn |
| ★★☆ | ★☆☆ |

Muscles used

Arms
Chest
Glutes

Glutes

| Flexibility | Flexibility |
| ★☆☆ | ★☆☆ |

🕐 **Keep at it for 5–10 minutes**

EXOTIC CHEST LIFT

Swivel your bodies to form an X shape and explore exciting side-entry angles.

They tense their chest while supporting their upper body weight

They fire up their glutes to thrust back and forth at this perpendicular angle

They can reciprocate their lover's movement to engage their glutes

FOOT PRESS PASSION

They can take charge by pulling your foot into their chest. You enjoy the dramatic tension of them leaning over you, knowing you could push them away at any moment.

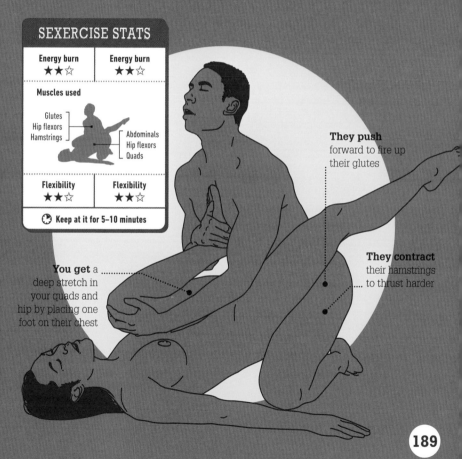

SEXERCISE STATS

Energy burn ★★☆	Energy burn ★★☆

Muscles used

Glutes
Hip flexors
Hamstrings

Abdominals
Hip flexors
Quads

Flexibility ★★☆	Flexibility ★★☆

🕐 Keep at it for 5–10 minutes

They push forward to fire up their glutes

They contract their hamstrings to thrust harder

You get a deep stretch in your quads and hip by placing one foot on their chest

SULTRY SHOULDER PRESS

They lean back seductively while maintaining intense eye contact—an ideal opportunity for attentive clitoral stimulation.

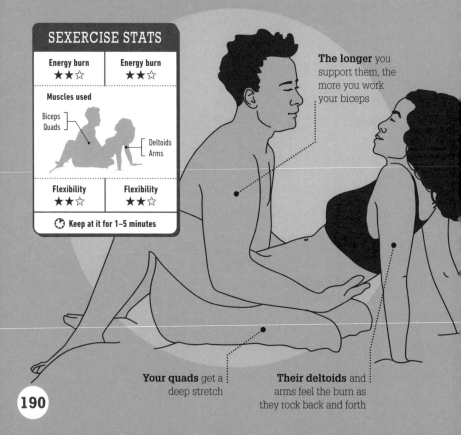

SEXERCISE STATS

Energy burn	Energy burn
★★☆	★★☆

Muscles used

Biceps
Quads

Deltoids
Arms

Flexibility	Flexibility
★★☆	★★☆

🕐 **Keep at it for 1–5 minutes**

The longer you support them, the more you work your biceps

Your quads get a deep stretch

Their deltoids and arms feel the burn as they rock back and forth

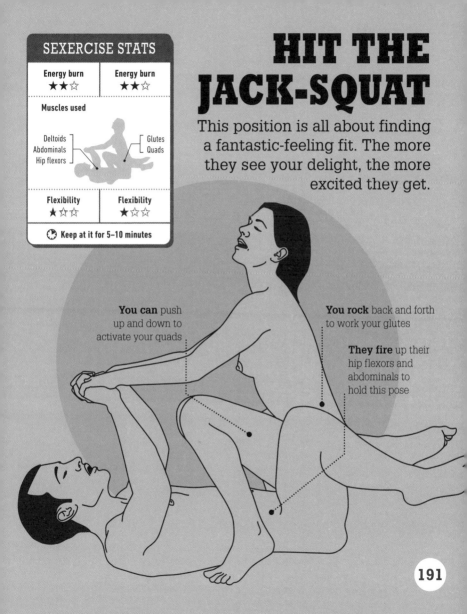

HIT THE JACK-SQUAT

This position is all about finding a fantastic-feeling fit. The more they see your delight, the more excited they get.

You can push up and down to activate your quads

You rock back and forth to work your glutes

They fire up their hip flexors and abdominals to hold this pose

191

SHOULDER SHUDDER

For seriously sensuous sex, pay special attention to their neck and shoulders: kiss, blow, and lick to make them quiver with delight.

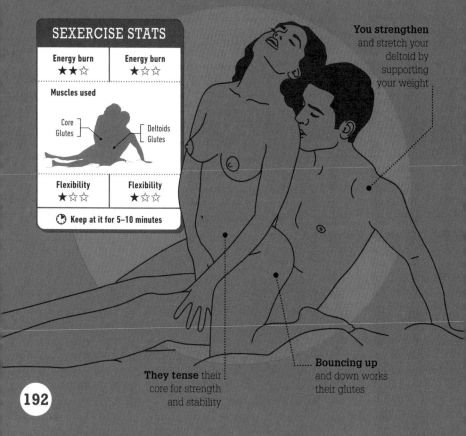

SEXERCISE STATS

Energy burn ★★☆	Energy burn ★☆☆
Muscles used	
Core / Glutes	Deltoids / Glutes
Flexibility ★☆☆	Flexibility ★☆☆

🕑 Keep at it for 5–10 minutes

You strengthen and stretch your deltoid by supporting your weight

They tense their core for strength and stability

Bouncing up and down works their glutes

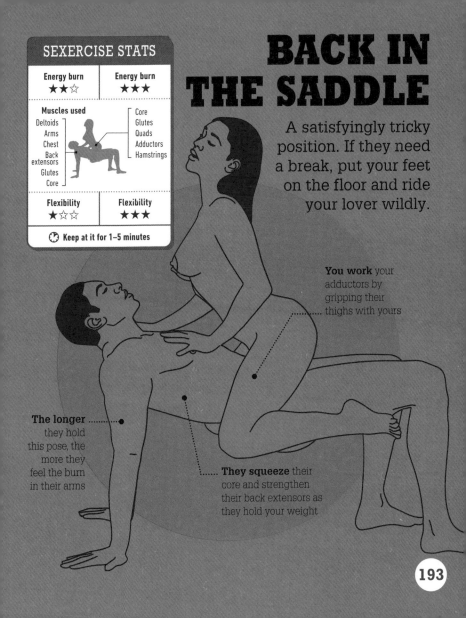

BACK IN THE SADDLE

A satisfyingly tricky position. If they need a break, put your feet on the floor and ride your lover wildly.

SEXERCISE STATS

Energy burn	Energy burn
★★☆	★★★

Muscles used

Deltoids
Arms
Chest
Back extensors
Glutes
Core

⎡ Core
⎢ Glutes
⎢ Quads
⎢ Adductors
⎣ Hamstrings

Flexibility	Flexibility
★☆☆	★★★

🕐 Keep at it for 1–5 minutes

You work your adductors by gripping their thighs with yours

The longer they hold this pose, the more they feel the burn in their arms

They squeeze their core and strengthen their back extensors as they hold your weight

CORE KILLER

Your lover clasps your body between their knees and you call the shots. You can heat it up by leaning forward slowly so you both see more of the action.

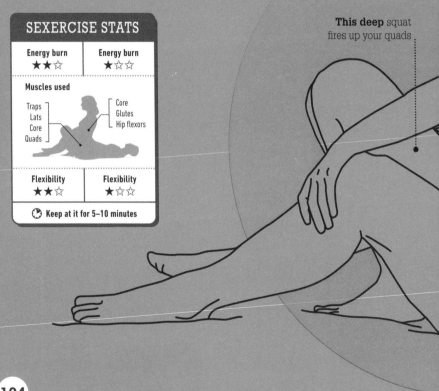

SEXERCISE STATS

Energy burn ★★☆	Energy burn ★☆☆

Muscles used

Traps
Lats
Core
Quads

Core
Glutes
Hip flexors

Flexibility ★★☆	Flexibility ★☆☆

🕐 Keep at it for 5–10 minutes

This deep squat fires up your quads

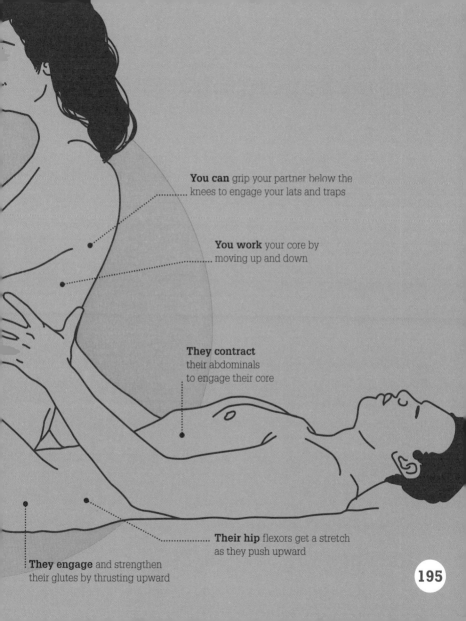

You can grip your partner below the knees to engage your lats and traps

You work your core by moving up and down

They contract their abdominals to engage their core

Their hip flexors get a stretch as they push upward

They engage and strengthen their glutes by thrusting upward

195

PEAK OF PLEASURE

When your lover is on top, lift your pelvis and thrust in midair. Excellent for eye contact and ensuring shudders of pleasure.

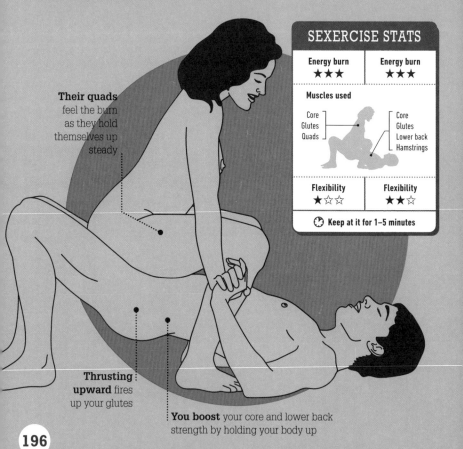

Their quads feel the burn as they hold themselves up steady

Thrusting upward fires up your glutes

You boost your core and lower back strength by holding your body up

SEXERCISE STATS

Energy burn	Energy burn
★★★	★★★

Muscles used

Core	Core
Glutes	Glutes
Quads	Lower back
	Hamstrings

Flexibility	Flexibility
★☆☆	★★☆

🕐 Keep at it for 1–5 minutes

SQUEEZE TO PLEASE

Your lover hangs their legs off the edge of the bed and clasps you tightly between their thighs. You bump your buttocks up and down to bring you both to climax.

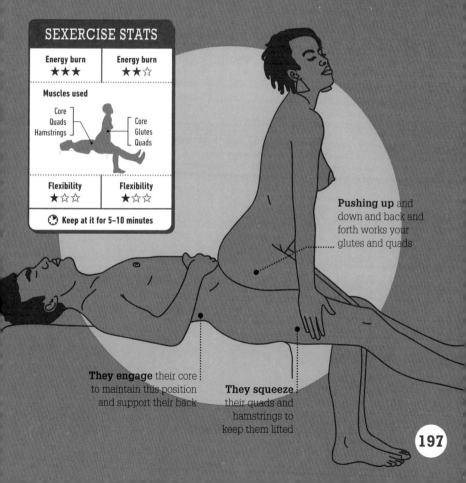

SEXERCISE STATS

Energy burn ★★★	Energy burn ★★☆

Muscles used

Core
Quads
Hamstrings

Core
Glutes
Quads

Flexibility ★☆☆	Flexibility ★☆☆

🕐 **Keep at it for 5–10 minutes**

Pushing up and down and back and forth works your glutes and quads

They engage their core to maintain this position and support their back

They squeeze their quads and hamstrings to keep them lifted

THIGH THRILLS

Arch your back provocatively and let them sink deeply into you. Try sustaining eye contact for an emotionally charged intensity.

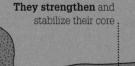
They strengthen and stabilize their core

You engage your core by tensing your deep abdominals and drawing up your lower spine

You squeeze your adductors to strengthen your hips

LOVERS' SQUEEZE

They wrap their legs around you and let you take the lead. You enjoy the firm grip of their thighs while giving their buttock a cheeky squeeze.

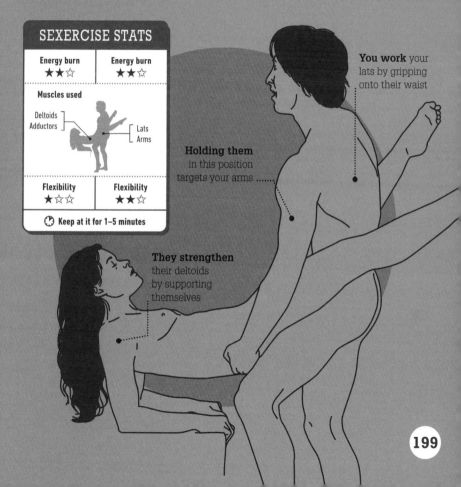

SEXERCISE STATS

Energy burn	Energy burn
★★☆	★★☆

Muscles used

Deltoids
Adductors

Lats
Arms

Flexibility	Flexibility
★☆☆	★★☆

🕑 Keep at it for 1–5 minutes

You work your lats by gripping onto their waist

Holding them in this position targets your arms

They strengthen their deltoids by supporting themselves

LUSTY LEG UP

Interlock your legs and
clasp each other close.
Seal the sensuality
with a lingering kiss.

SEXERCISE STATS

Energy burn	Energy burn
★★☆	★★☆

Muscles used

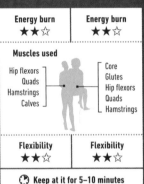

Hip flexors	Core
Quads	Glutes
Hamstrings	Hip flexors
Calves	Quads
	Hamstrings

Flexibility	Flexibility
★★☆	★★☆

🕐 **Keep at it for 5–10 minutes**

Rotating their thigh outward boosts the mobility in their hips

They strengthen their quads and hamstrings by standing on one leg

They push up from their toes to strengthen their calves

DEEP SQUAT DESIRE

You lean back against a wall and make them work hard.
When their thighs can no longer take the burn, they can
stand up straight and thrust freely to the finish.

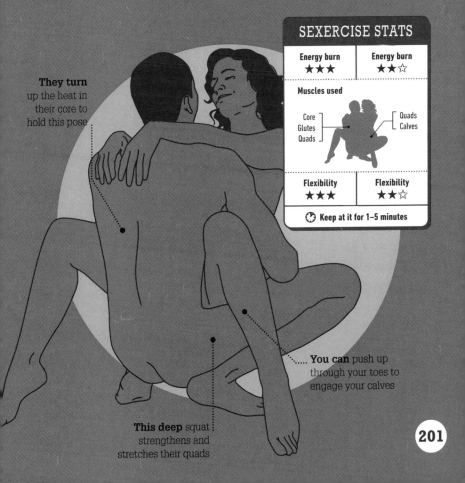

They turn up the heat in their core to hold this pose

SEXERCISE STATS

Energy burn	Energy burn
★★★	★★☆

Muscles used

Core
Glutes
Quads

Quads
Calves

Flexibility	Flexibility
★★★	★★☆

🕑 Keep at it for 1–5 minutes

You can push up through your toes to engage your calves

This deep squat strengthens and stretches their quads

201

STIFF COMPETITION

Your partner creates a firm table with their body, and you slot yourself on top. Competitive couples, keep it going until there's a winner.

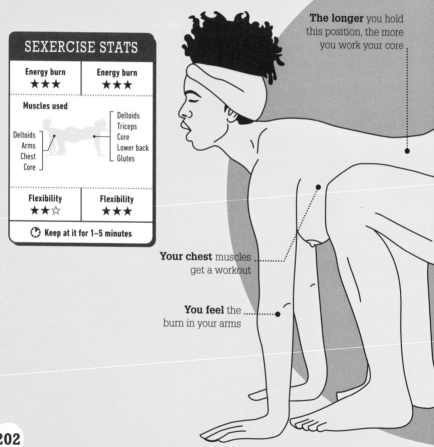

SEXERCISE STATS

Energy burn ★★★	Energy burn ★★★
Muscles used	
Deltoids Arms Chest Core	Deltoids Triceps Core Lower back Glutes
Flexibility ★★☆	Flexibility ★★★

⏱ Keep at it for 1–5 minutes

The longer you hold this position, the more you work your core

Your chest muscles get a workout

You feel the burn in your arms

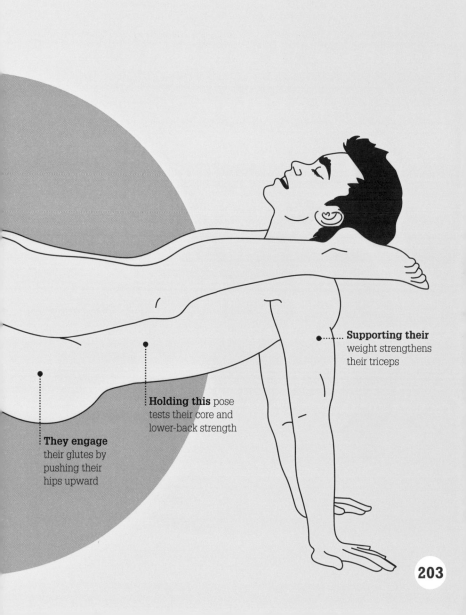

Supporting their weight strengthens their triceps

Holding this pose tests their core and lower-back strength

They engage their glutes by pushing their hips upward

203

LIFT AND PLUNGE

Your lover grabs your buttocks and enters deeply.
Bringing your knees to your chest creates a tight fit,
so you both feel every sensation intensely.

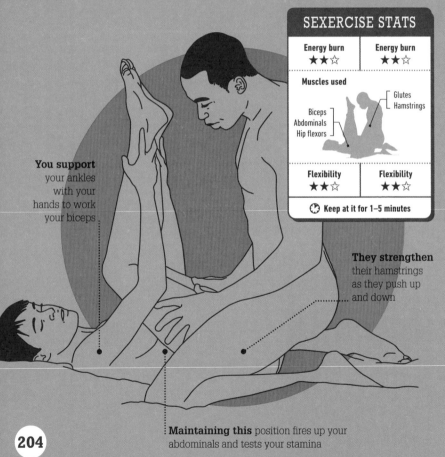

You support your ankles with your hands to work your biceps

They strengthen their hamstrings as they push up and down

Maintaining this position fires up your abdominals and tests your stamina

SEXERCISE STATS

Energy burn	Energy burn
★★☆	★★☆

Muscles used

Biceps
Abdominals
Hip flexors

Glutes
Hamstrings

Flexibility	Flexibility
★★☆	★★☆

🕐 **Keep at it for 1–5 minutes**

CENSATIONAL SWING

Sweep them away in this striking standing position. Your muscle power makes your lover melt.

Keeping them up strengthens your lats and arms

They tense their biceps and lats to stay in this position

You work your quads and hamstrings to lift them into position and hold them up

SEXERCISE STATS

Energy burn ★★★	Energy burn ★★☆
Muscles used	
Arms Lats Core Hamstrings Quads	Biceps Lats Core
Flexibility ★★☆	Flexibility ★★★
🕑 Keep at it for 1–5 minutes	

205

BRAWN MEETS BEAUTY

They hold you up in a feat of strength. You lean back against a wall to reward them with a view of your chest.

SEXERCISE STATS

Energy burn	Energy burn
★★★	★★★

Muscles used

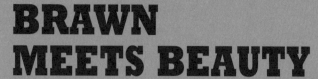

Traps	Core
Lats	Glutes
Core	Adductors
Glutes	Hamstrings
Quads	

Flexibility	Flexibility
★★☆	★★☆

🕐 Keep at it for 1–5 minutes

You grip their waist with your thighs to work your adductors

They tense their core and lats to stabilize themselves

Lifting you into position and staying steady strengthens their quads

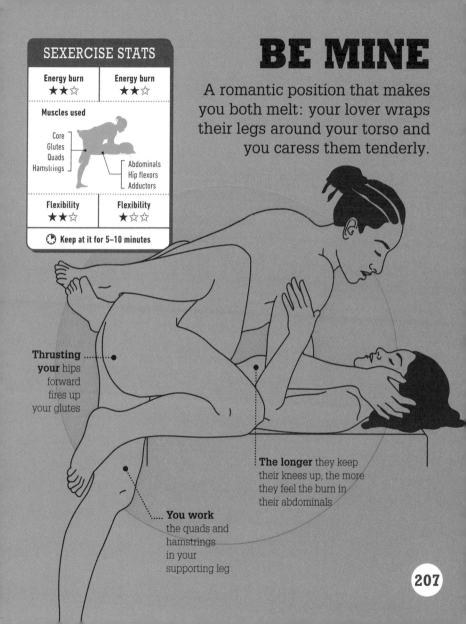

SEXERCISE STATS

Energy burn	Energy burn
★★☆	★★☆

Muscles used

Core
Glutes
Quads
Hamstrings

Abdominals
Hip flexors
Adductors

Flexibility	Flexibility
★★☆	★☆☆

🕐 Keep at it for 5–10 minutes

BE MINE

A romantic position that makes you both melt: your lover wraps their legs around your torso and you caress them tenderly.

Thrusting your hips forward fires up your glutes

The longer they keep their knees up, the more they feel the burn in their abdominals

You work the quads and hamstrings in your supporting leg

HELPING H■ND

Interlace your fingers and look into each other's eyes, then break free and get your hands dirty by using them to maximize your pleasure.

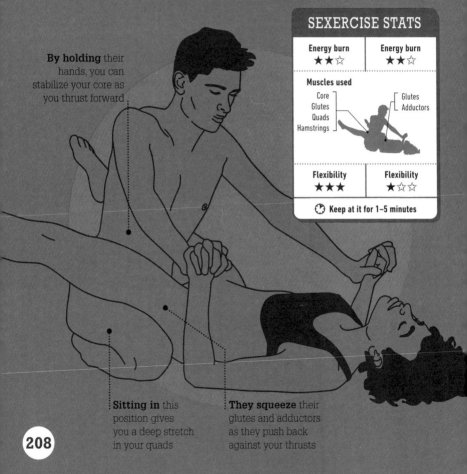

By holding their hands, you can stabilize your core as you thrust forward

Sitting in this position gives you a deep stretch in your quads

They squeeze their glutes and adductors as they push back against your thrusts

SEXERCISE STATS

Energy burn ★★☆	Energy burn ★★☆

Muscles used

Core
Glutes
Quads
Hamstrings

Glutes
Adductors

Flexibility ★★★	Flexibility ★☆☆

🕐 Keep at it for 1–5 minutes

REAR-ENTRY

A wheelbarrow, but not as you know it:
they straddle you between their legs to
create sparks of fizzing friction.

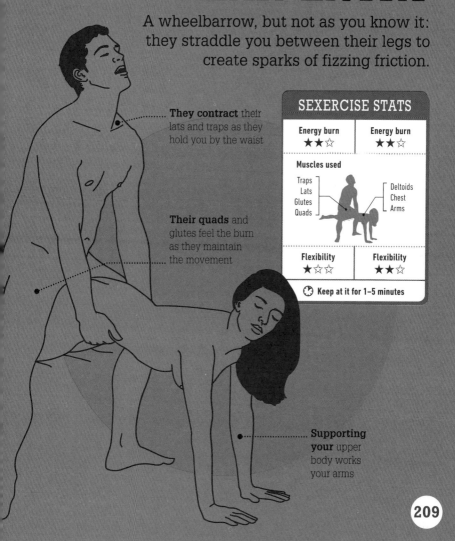

They contract their
lats and traps as they
hold you by the waist

Their quads and
glutes feel the burn
as they maintain
the movement

SEXERCISE STATS

Energy burn ★★☆	Energy burn ★★☆

Muscles used

Traps
Lats
Glutes
Quads

Deltoids
Chest
Arms

Flexibility ★☆☆	Flexibility ★★☆

🕑 Keep at it for 1–5 minutes

**Supporting
your** upper
body works
your arms

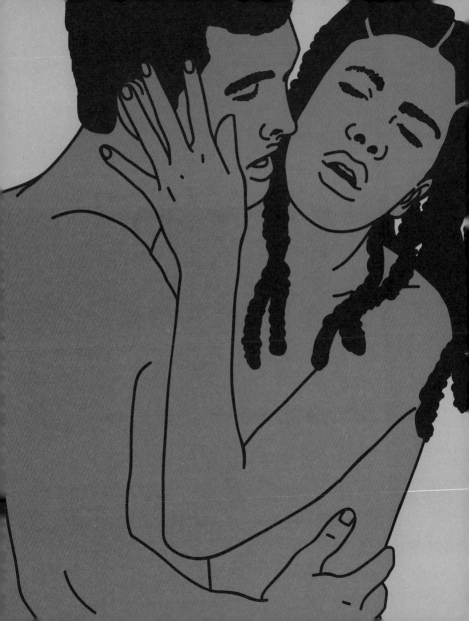

"A LOVING PAIR
BECOME BLIND WITH
passion
IN THE HEAT OF
CONGRESS"

THE KAMA SUTRA

LUSTY LOTUS

All the intensity of ardent eye contact, but with the sexy barrier of your crossed legs. They find your suppleness super arousing.

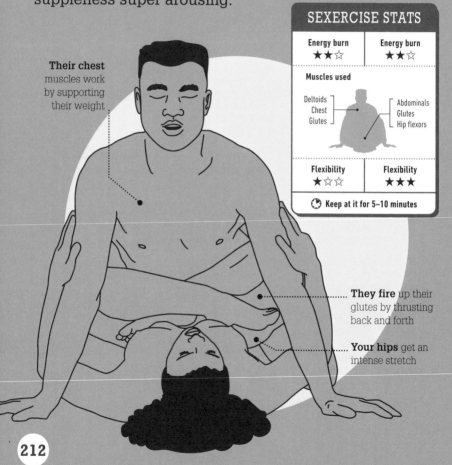

Their chest muscles work by supporting their weight

They fire up their glutes by thrusting back and forth

Your hips get an intense stretch

SEXERCISE STATS

Energy burn	Energy burn
★★☆	★★☆

Muscles used

Deltoids
Chest
Glutes

Abdominals
Glutes
Hip flexors

Flexibility	Flexibility
★☆☆	★★★

🕐 Keep at it for 5–10 minutes

FOLD AND FONDLE

Your lover bends over and shows you exactly where they want you. Spooning from behind leaves you both feeling close and connected.

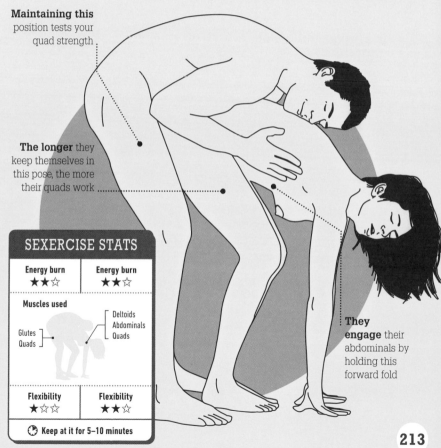

Maintaining this position tests your quad strength

The longer they keep themselves in this pose, the more their quads work

They engage their abdominals by holding this forward fold

SEXERCISE STATS

Energy burn ★★☆	Energy burn ★★☆

Muscles used

Glutes Quads

Deltoids Abdominals Quads

Flexibility ★☆☆	Flexibility ★★☆

⏱ **Keep at it for 5–10 minutes**

213

THE STRONGMAN

Add muscle to your missionary. You show off your tricep strength, while your lover wraps their legs around you and voices their appreciation.

Thrusting up and down fires up your glutes

Squeezing their hips up and down activates their glutes and core

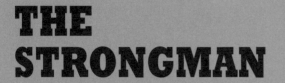

SEXERCISE STATS

Energy burn	Energy burn
★★★	★☆☆

Muscles used

Deltoids
Arms
Chest
Core
Lower back
Glutes

Core
Glutes
Adductors

Flexibility	Flexibility
★☆☆	★★☆

🕐 **Keep at it for 1–5 minutes**

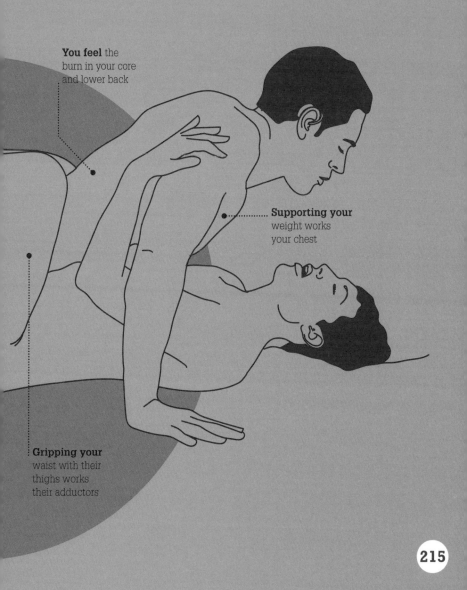

You feel the burn in your core and lower back

Supporting your weight works your chest

Gripping your waist with their thighs works their adductors

215

SEXY HALF SPLITS

Your partner strokes your leg seductively and thrusts gently to build up arousal slowly. You'll reap all the benefits of prolonged stimulation.

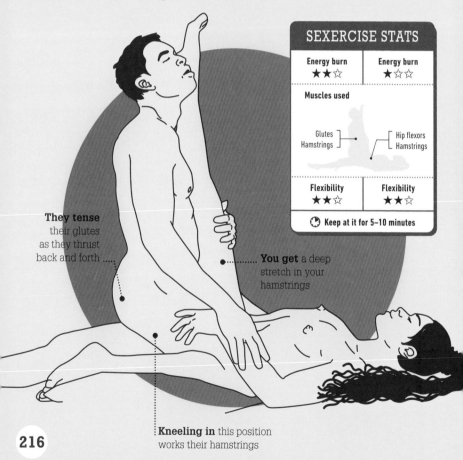

SEXERCISE STATS

Energy burn	Energy burn
★★☆	★☆☆

Muscles used

Glutes
Hamstrings

Hip flexors
Hamstrings

Flexibility	Flexibility
★★☆	★★☆

⏱ Keep at it for 5–10 minutes

They tense their glutes as they thrust back and forth

You get a deep stretch in your hamstrings

Kneeling in this position works their hamstrings

ROCK BOTTOM

Your lover lifts their leg and lets you in. This position gets top marks for g-spot stimulation and screams for some anal attention.

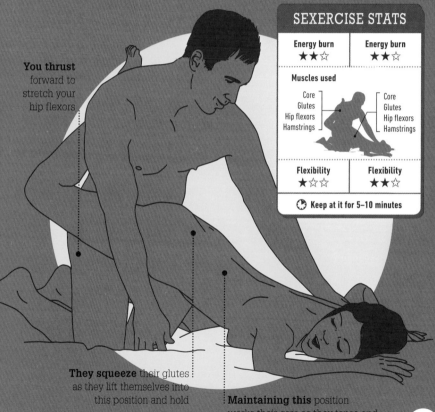

You thrust forward to stretch your hip flexors

SEXERCISE STATS

Energy burn	Energy burn
★★☆	★★☆

Muscles used

Core Glutes Hip flexors Hamstrings		Core Glutes Hip flexors Hamstrings

Flexibility	Flexibility
★☆☆	★★☆

🕑 **Keep at it for 5–10 minutes**

They squeeze their glutes as they lift themselves into this position and hold

Maintaining this position works their core as they tense and push back against your thrusts

HEIGHTS OF SEXTASY

All the here-and-now kinkiness of a standing position but without the burn for your arms.

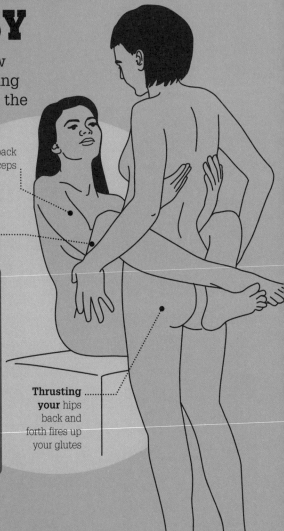

Gripping your back works their biceps

They strengthen their adductors as they wrap their legs around your waist

Thrusting your hips back and forth fires up your glutes

SEXERCISE STATS

Energy burn ★★☆	Energy burn ★☆☆
Muscles used	
Biceps Core Glutes Adductors	Glutes
Flexibility ★☆☆	Flexibility ★☆☆
🕐 Keep at it for 5–10 minutes	

AT ARM'S LENGTH

When your arousal is at its peak, keep each other at a tantalizing distance and rock back and forth. Start off slowly, then pick up the pace for a fierce climax.

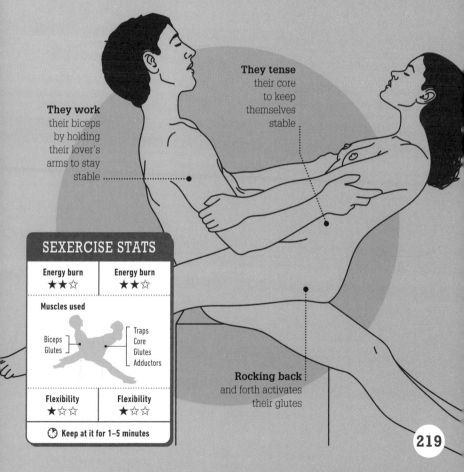

They tense their core to keep themselves stable

They work their biceps by holding their lover's arms to stay stable

Rocking back and forth activates their glutes

SEXERCISE STATS

Energy burn	Energy burn
★★☆	★★☆

Muscles used

Biceps
Glutes

Traps
Core
Glutes
Adductors

Flexibility	Flexibility
★☆☆	★☆☆

🕑 Keep at it for 1–5 minutes

SINGLE-HANDED

This position is a dazzling display of sexual dexterity. You balance on one arm so they can enter you at a sensational side angle.

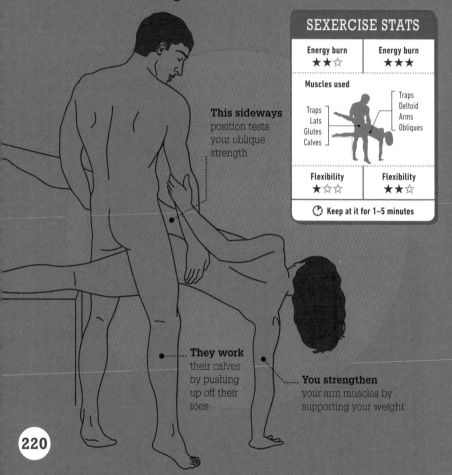

This sideways position tests your oblique strength

SEXERCISE STATS

Energy burn ★★☆	Energy burn ★★★

Muscles used

Traps
Lats
Glutes
Calves

Traps
Deltoid
Arms
Obliques

Flexibility ★☆☆	Flexibility ★★☆

🕐 **Keep at it for 1–5 minutes**

They work their calves by pushing up off their toes

You strengthen your arm muscles by supporting your weight

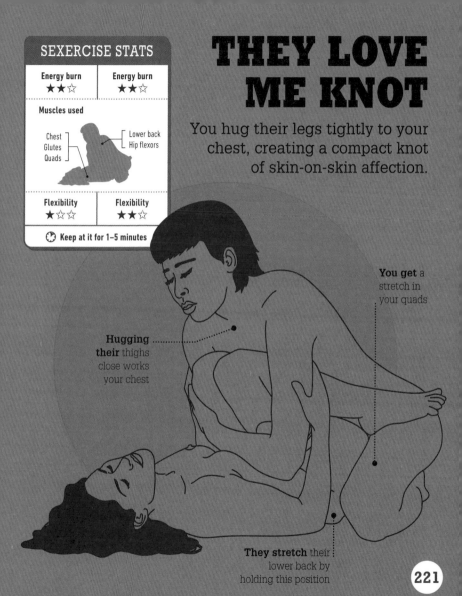

SEXERCISE STATS

Energy burn	Energy burn
★★☆	★★☆

Muscles used

Chest
Glutes
Quads

Lower back
Hip flexors

Flexibility	Flexibility
★☆☆	★★☆

🕐 Keep at it for 1–5 minutes

THEY LOVE ME KNOT

You hug their legs tightly to your chest, creating a compact knot of skin-on-skin affection.

You get a stretch in your quads

Hugging their thighs close works your chest

They stretch their lower back by holding this position

221

LEAN OF LOVE

All the face-to-face intimacy of missionary with none of the mundanity: melt into your lover's limbs and get swept away.

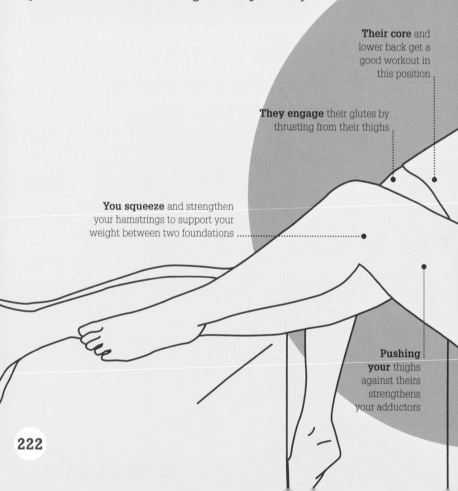

Their core and lower back get a good workout in this position

They engage their glutes by thrusting from their thighs

You squeeze and strengthen your hamstrings to support your weight between two foundations

Pushing your thighs against theirs strengthens your adductors

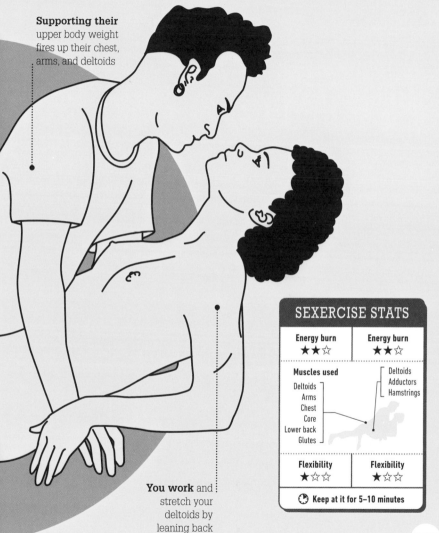

Supporting their upper body weight fires up their chest, arms, and deltoids

You work and stretch your deltoids by leaning back

SEXERCISE STATS

Energy burn	Energy burn
★★☆	★★☆

Muscles used	
Deltoids Arms Chest Core Lower back Glutes	Deltoids Adductors Hamstrings

Flexibility	Flexibility
★☆☆	★☆☆

🕐 **Keep at it for 5–10 minutes**

223

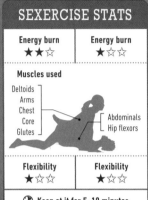

SEXERCISE STATS

Energy burn ★★☆	Energy burn ★☆☆
Muscles used	

Deltoids
Arms
Chest
Core
Glutes

Abdominals
Hip flexors

Flexibility ★☆☆	Flexibility ★☆☆

🕐 Keep at it for 5–10 minutes

CORE VALUES

Raise your legs to let them enter deeply. They can turn up the orgasmic energy by rubbing your clitoris.

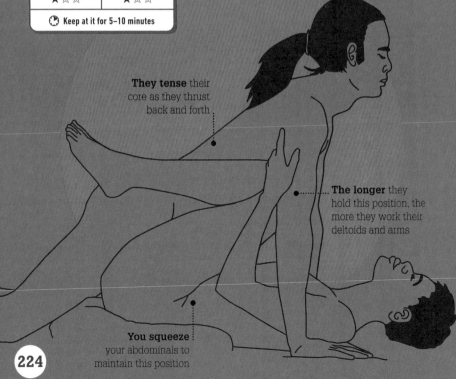

They tense their core as they thrust back and forth

The longer they hold this position, the more they work their deltoids and arms

You squeeze your abdominals to maintain this position

224

SLIDE TO SATISFY

They sit on your lap, then slide their hands down your legs so you can slip in easily.

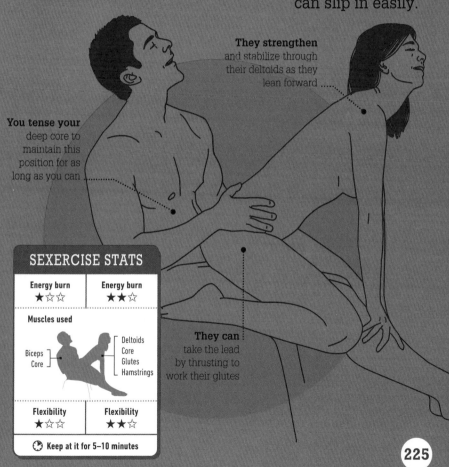

They strengthen and stabilize through their deltoids as they lean forward

You tense your deep core to maintain this position for as long as you can

They can take the lead by thrusting to work their glutes

SEXERCISE STATS

Energy burn ★☆☆	Energy burn ★★☆

Muscles used

Biceps
Core

Deltoids
Core
Glutes
Hamstrings

Flexibility ★☆☆	Flexibility ★★☆

🕑 Keep at it for 5–10 minutes

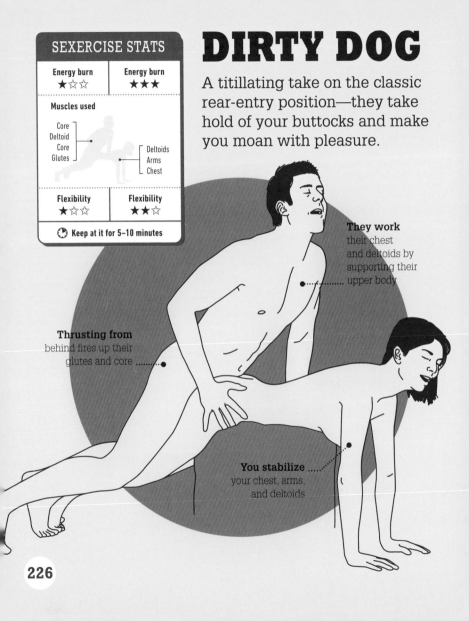

DIRTY DOG

A titillating take on the classic rear-entry position—they take hold of your buttocks and make you moan with pleasure.

SEXERCISE STATS

Energy burn	Energy burn
★☆☆	★★★

Muscles used

Core
Deltoid
Core
Glutes

Deltoids
Arms
Chest

Flexibility	Flexibility
★☆☆	★★☆

🕐 Keep at it for 5–10 minutes

They work their chest and deltoids by supporting their upper body

Thrusting from behind fires up their glutes and core

You stabilize your chest, arms, and deltoids

226

X-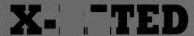TED

You push your thighs against theirs to make them deliciously tight. Lean in for a loving kiss, or lie back and enjoy the ride.

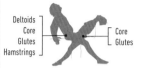

SEXERCISE STATS

Energy burn	Energy burn
★☆☆	★★★

Muscles used

Deltoids
Core
Glutes
Hamstrings

Core
Glutes

Flexibility	Flexibility
★☆☆	★★☆

🕐 Keep at it for 5–10 minutes

You tense your abdominals while maintaining the movement to strengthen your core

They work their glutes by reciprocating your thrusts

You engage your hamstrings by thrusting through your pelvis

227

LYRE PLAYER

Drape your legs over your lover's chest and let them pluck your strings until they hear you moan. Perfect for seriously sensual lovemaking.

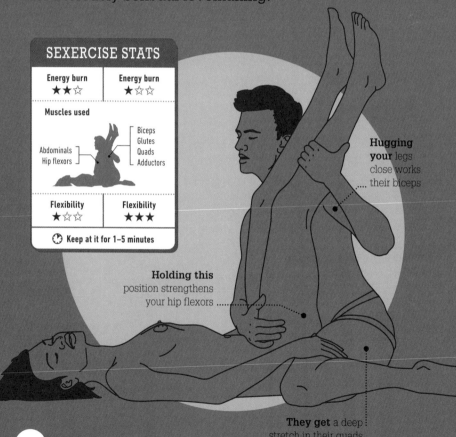

SEXERCISE STATS

Energy burn	Energy burn
★★☆	★☆☆

Muscles used

Abdominals
Hip flexors

Biceps
Glutes
Quads
Adductors

Flexibility	Flexibility
★☆☆	★★★

🕑 Keep at it for 1–5 minutes

Hugging your legs close works their biceps

Holding this position strengthens your hip flexors

They get a deep stretch in their quads and adductors

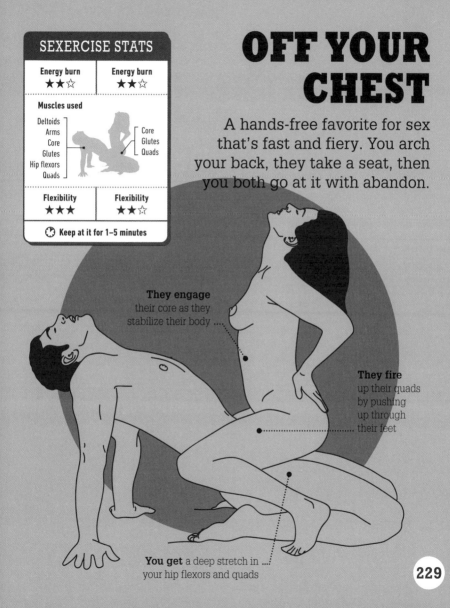

OFF YOUR CHEST

A hands-free favorite for sex that's fast and fiery. You arch your back, they take a seat, then you both go at it with abandon.

SEXERCISE STATS

Energy burn	Energy burn
★★☆	★★☆

Muscles used

Deltoids
Arms
Core
Glutes
Hip flexors
Quads

Core
Glutes
Quads

Flexibility	Flexibility
★★★	★★☆

🕐 Keep at it for 1–5 minutes

They engage their core as they stabilize their body

They fire up their quads by pushing up through their feet

You get a deep stretch in your hip flexors and quads

229

BE MY VALENTINE

A winner for slow and sumptuous lovemaking: their hands can roam all over your body, making you feel truly seduced.

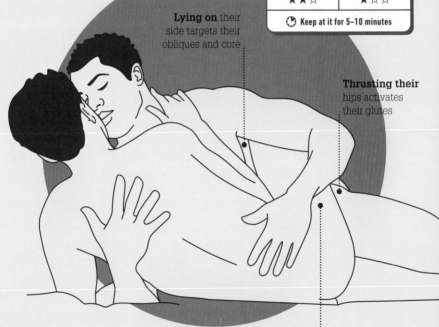

Lying on their side targets their obliques and core

Thrusting their hips activates their glutes

You work your hamstrings by squeezing your legs behind them

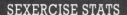

Energy burn	Energy burn
★★☆	★★☆

Muscles used

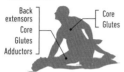

Back extensors
Core
Glutes
Adductors

Core
Glutes

Flexibility	Flexibility
★★☆	★☆☆

🕐 **Keep at it for 1–5 minutes**

TIP-TOP FORM

You might be on top, but it's your lover calling the shots. They tell you exactly what to do to make them writhe with pleasure.

You strengthen your glutes by thrusting back and forth

They work their core and back hard to maintain this position ..

Squeezing your hips with their legs activates their adductors

231

GLUTE CAMP

Enjoy the eroticism of this dramatic position. You open wide and surrender to the power of their passion.

They work their deltoids by holding this position

Lifting your legs and holding them back strengthens your abdominals

They get a good stretch through their glutes and adductors

232

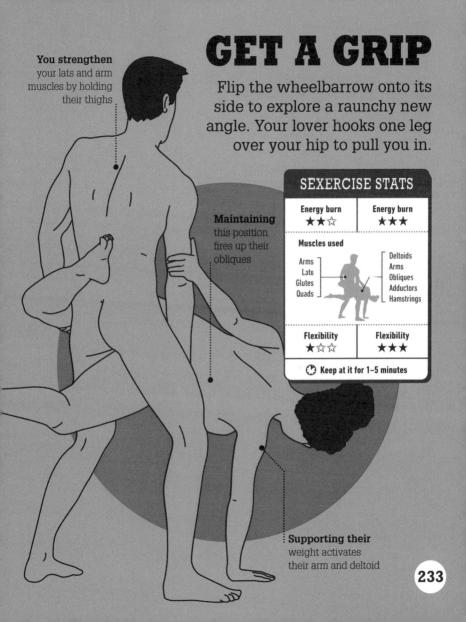

GET A GRIP

Flip the wheelbarrow onto its side to explore a raunchy new angle. Your lover hooks one leg over your hip to pull you in.

You strengthen your lats and arm muscles by holding their thighs

Maintaining this position fires up their obliques

Supporting their weight activates their arm and deltoid

SEXERCISE STATS

Energy burn	Energy burn
★★☆	★★★

Muscles used

Arms	Deltoids
Lats	Arms
Glutes	Obliques
Quads	Adductors
	Hamstrings

Flexibility	Flexibility
★☆☆	★★★

🕐 **Keep at it for 1–5 minutes**

233

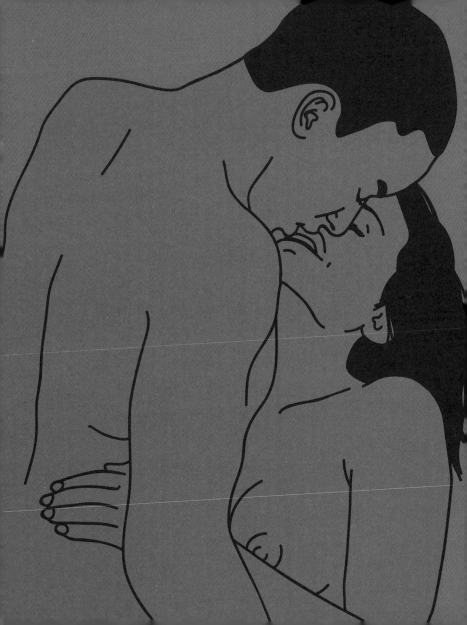

"**FASCINATED** **BY VARIOUS** **FORMS OF** *kissing* **THEY DELIGHT IN THE** **CLOSEST** *embraces*"

THE ANANGA RANGA

LADY OF PLEASURE

You're face to face but kept tantalizingly apart by your raised feet. You lie back and crosses your ankles, then they push themselves into you powerfully.

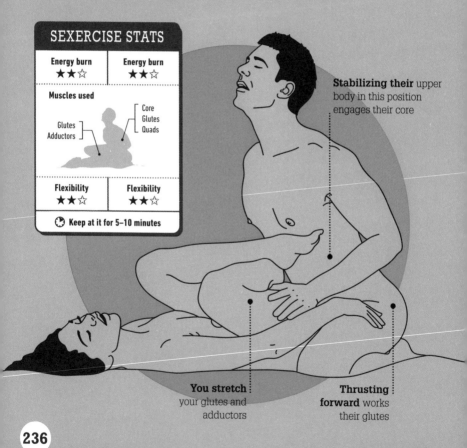

SEXERCISE STATS

Energy burn	Energy burn
★★☆	★★☆

Muscles used

Glutes
Adductors

Core
Glutes
Quads

Flexibility	Flexibility
★★☆	★★☆

🕐 Keep at it for 5–10 minutes

Stabilizing their upper body in this position engages their core

You stretch your glutes and adductors

Thrusting forward works their glutes

WALLFLOWER

For moments of burning desire—your lover wraps themselves around your torso, you support them against the wall, and you both yield to your yearnings.

Holding them up strengthens your lats, traps, and core

They work their adductors by gripping your hips with their thighs

Lifting them into position fires up your glutes, quads, and hamstrings

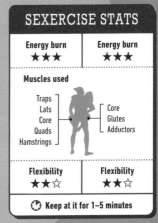

SEXERCISE STATS

Energy burn ★★★	Energy burn ★★★
Muscles used	
Traps Lats Core Quads Hamstrings	Core Glutes Adductors
Flexibility ★★☆	Flexibility ★★☆
🕑 Keep at it for 1–5 minutes	

TURN THE TABLES

Your love invites you to sit at their table and serves up your favorite dish. The enticing view of your beautiful buttocks is the reward for all their hard work.

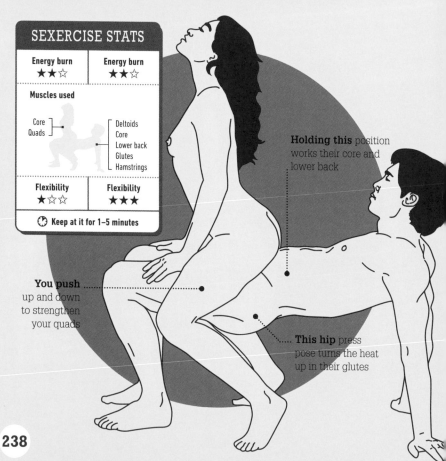

SEXERCISE STATS

Energy burn	Energy burn
★★☆	★★☆

Muscles used

Core
Quads

- Deltoids
- Core
- Lower back
- Glutes
- Hamstrings

Flexibility	Flexibility
★☆☆	★★★

🕐 Keep at it for 1–5 minutes

Holding this position works their core and lower back

You push up and down to strengthen your quads

This hip press pose turns the heat up in their glutes

SENSATIONAL SPLITS

If your partner is super supple, lean in and push their leg toward them for a show-stopping stretch. Sliding your fingers up and down will make them shudder.

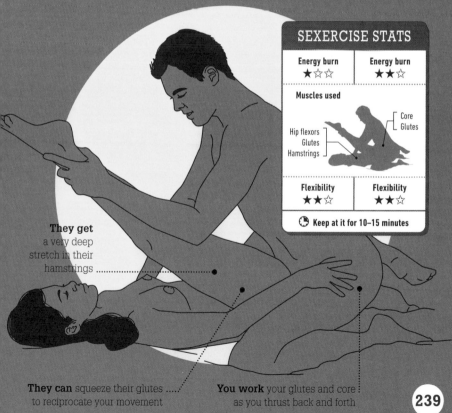

SEXERCISE STATS

Energy burn ★☆☆	Energy burn ★★☆
Muscles used	
Hip flexors, Glutes, Hamstrings — Core, Glutes	
Flexibility ★★☆	Flexibility ★★☆

🕑 Keep at it for 10–15 minutes

They get a very deep stretch in their hamstrings

They can squeeze their glutes to reciprocate your movement

You work your glutes and core as you thrust back and forth

239

POWER PLAY

You lie back and relinquish all control. They keep you on the edge by mixing frenzied bounces with tantalizingly slow strokes.

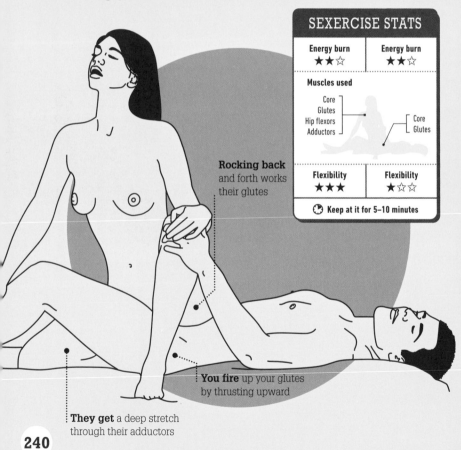

Rocking back and forth works their glutes

SEXERCISE STATS

Energy burn	Energy burn
★★☆	★★☆

Muscles used

Core
Glutes
Hip flexors
Adductors

Core
Glutes

Flexibility	Flexibility
★★★	★☆☆

🕐 **Keep at it for 5–10 minutes**

You fire up your glutes by thrusting upward

They get a deep stretch through their adductors

LEARNING CURVE

Exquisite and lust-quenching in equal measure:
you arch your back and rest your toes on their calves
while they hold you firmly by the waist.

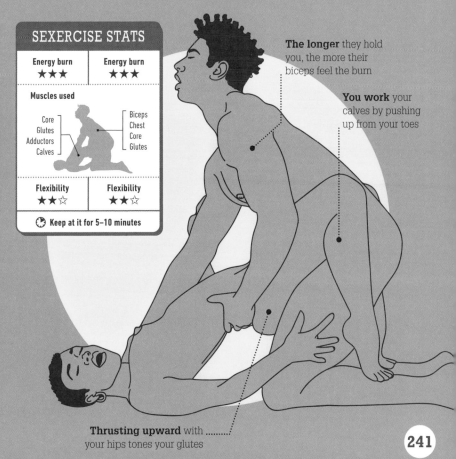

SEXERCISE STATS

Energy burn	Energy burn
★★★	★★★

Muscles used

Core	Biceps
Glutes	Chest
Adductors	Core
Calves	Glutes

Flexibility	Flexibility
★★☆	★★☆

🕐 Keep at it for 5–10 minutes

The longer they hold
you, the more their
biceps feel the burn

You work your
calves by pushing
up from your toes

Thrusting upward with
your hips tones your glutes

G___CH ___'D G___O__

Hold tight and lose yourselves in your lovemaking. You're excellently placed to spin yourself around and experiment with any angle of entry.

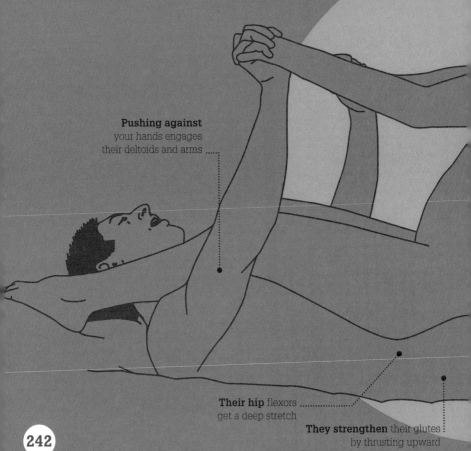

Pushing against your hands engages their deltoids and arms

Their hip flexors get a deep stretch

They strengthen their glutes by thrusting upward

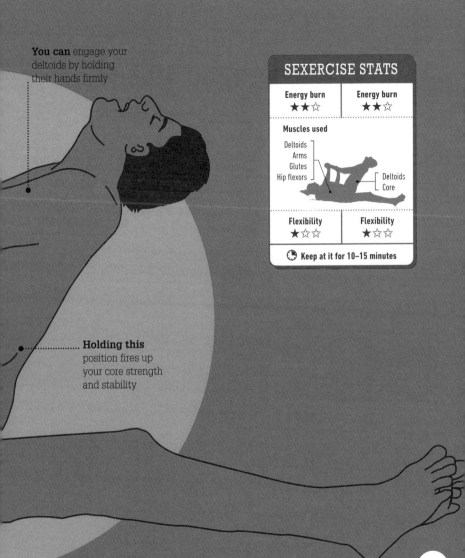

You can engage your deltoids by holding their hands firmly

Holding this position fires up your core strength and stability

SEXERCISE STATS

Energy burn ★★☆	Energy burn ★★☆
Muscles used	

Deltoids
Arms
Glutes
Hip flexors

Deltoids
Core

Flexibility ★☆☆	Flexibility ★☆☆

🕒 Keep at it for 10–15 minutes

TOUCH YOUR TOES

Your lover bends over as far as they can and teases you with a view of their beautiful buttocks.

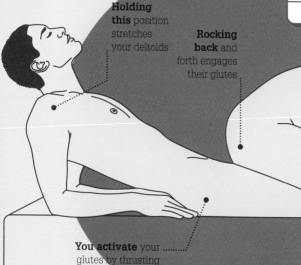

Holding this position stretches your deltoids

Rocking back and forth engages their glutes

You activate your glutes by thrusting your hips upward

244

PRESS MY BUTTONS

You press one foot against their stomach and the other over their shoulder. To prolong the passion, try swapping legs.

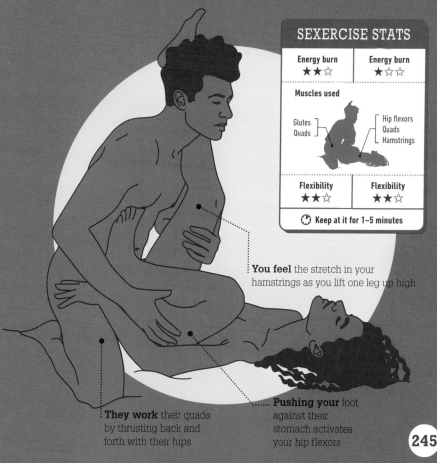

SEXERCISE STATS

Energy burn	Energy burn
★★☆	★☆☆

Muscles used

Glutes
Quads

Hip flexors
Quads
Hamstrings

Flexibility	Flexibility
★★☆	★★☆

🕐 Keep at it for 1–5 minutes

You feel the stretch in your hamstrings as you lift one leg up high

They work their quads by thrusting back and forth with their hips

Pushing your foot against their stomach activates your hip flexors

FORWARD BEND

A no-frills favorite for when you want to get down and dirty. You get onto all fours, and you both unleash your primal instincts.

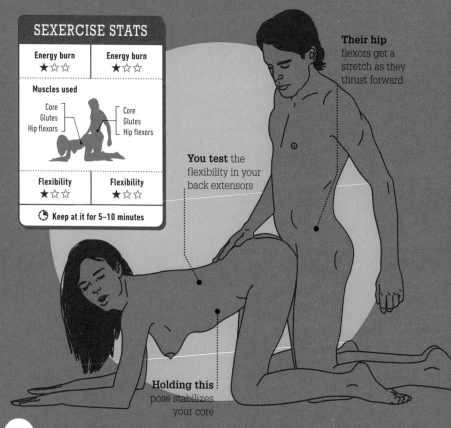

SEXERCISE STATS

Energy burn	Energy burn
★☆☆	★☆☆

Muscles used

Core
Glutes
Hip flexors

Core
Glutes
Hip flexors

Flexibility	Flexibility
★☆☆	★☆☆

🕑 **Keep at it for 5–10 minutes**

Their hip flexors get a stretch as they thrust forward

You test the flexibility in your back extensors

Holding this pose stabilizes your core

246

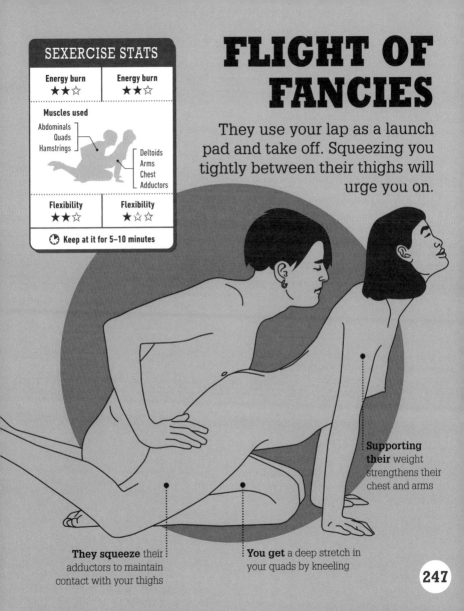

FLIGHT OF FANCIES

They use your lap as a launch pad and take off. Squeezing you tightly between their thighs will urge you on.

SEXERCISE STATS

Energy burn	Energy burn
★★☆	★★☆

Muscles used

Abdominals
Quads
Hamstrings

Deltoids
Arms
Chest
Adductors

Flexibility	Flexibility
★★☆	★☆☆

🕓 Keep at it for 5–10 minutes

Supporting their weight strengthens their chest and arms

They squeeze their adductors to maintain contact with your thighs

You get a deep stretch in your quads by kneeling

247

ROCKET LAUNCHER

One partner fires up their love rocket, while the other buckles up and lifts off for some out-of-this-world loving.

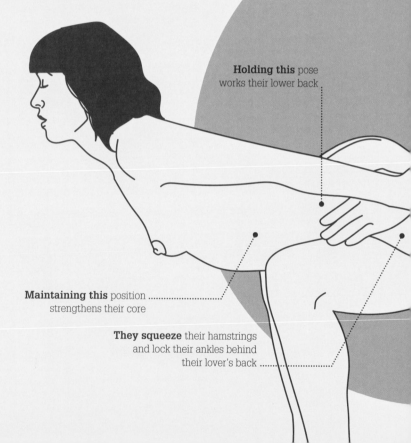

Holding this pose works their lower back

Maintaining this position strengthens their core

They squeeze their hamstrings and lock their ankles behind their lover's back

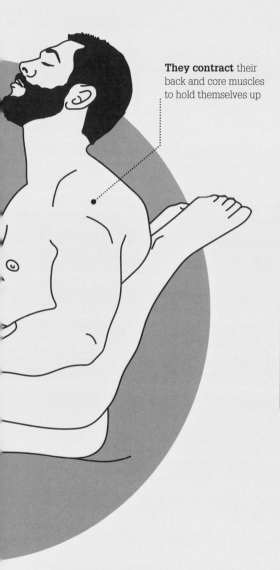

They contract their back and core muscles to hold themselves up

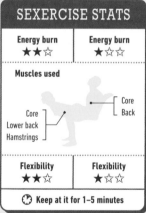

SEXERCISE STATS

Energy burn	Energy burn
★★☆	★☆☆

Muscles used

Core
Back

Core
Lower back
Hamstrings

Flexibility	Flexibility
★★☆	★☆☆

🕐 Keep at it for 1–5 minutes

249

LIFT OFF

Fire up your love engines and prepare to take flight. Your lover presses their hands into a wall to absorb the force of your thrusts.

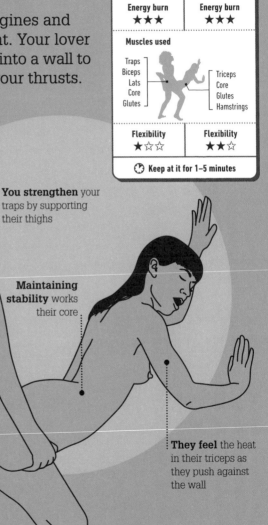

SEXERCISE STATS

Energy burn	Energy burn
★★★	★★★

Muscles used

Traps
Biceps
Lats
Core
Glutes

Triceps
Core
Glutes
Hamstrings

Flexibility	Flexibility
★☆☆	★★☆

🕐 Keep at it for 1–5 minutes

You strengthen your traps by supporting their thighs

Maintaining stability works their core

They feel the heat in their triceps as they push against the wall

250

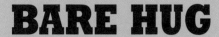

BARE HUG

When you're aching for skin contact, entwine yourselves in each other's arms and relish every touch.

They engage their chest by holding on tightly

Their biceps and chest work as they wrap their arms around their lover

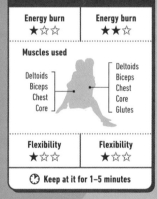

SEXERCISE STATS

Energy burn	Energy burn
★☆☆	★★☆

Muscles used

Deltoids
Biceps
Chest
Core

Deltoids
Biceps
Chest
Core
Glutes

Flexibility	Flexibility
★☆☆	★☆☆

🕐 Keep at it for 1–5 minutes

Pulsing up and down activates their glutes

251

WITHIN REACH

Hold each other just at arm's length and let the sexual tension build to the breaking point.

Maintaining this upright position engages their core

They work their lats by pulling their lover toward them

They work their glutes by moving back and forth

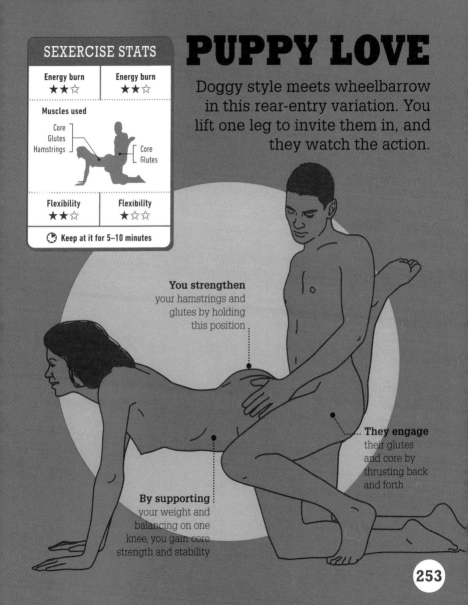

SEXERCISE STATS

Energy burn	Energy burn
★★☆	★★☆

Muscles used

Core
Glutes
Hamstrings

Core
Glutes

Flexibility	Flexibility
★★☆	★☆☆

🕐 Keep at it for 5–10 minutes

PUPPY LOVE

Doggy style meets wheelbarrow in this rear-entry variation. You lift one leg to invite them in, and they watch the action.

You strengthen
your hamstrings and glutes by holding this position

They engage
their glutes and core by thrusting back and forth

By supporting
your weight and balancing on one knee, you gain core strength and stability

BENCHWARMER

Side-entry sex that feels so casual, it's almost accidental: take a seat on your lover's bench and get a saucy surprise.

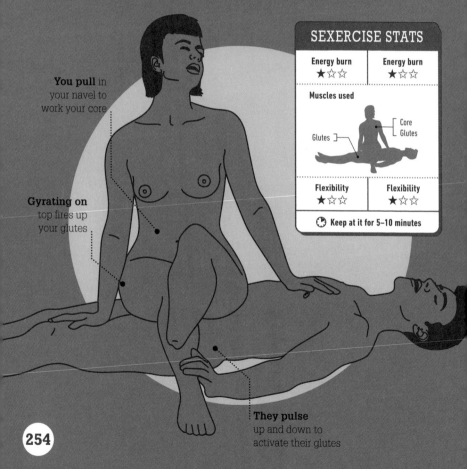

You pull in your navel to work your core

Gyrating on top fires up your glutes

They pulse up and down to activate their glutes

SEXERCISE STATS

Energy burn	Energy burn
★☆☆	★☆☆

Muscles used

Glutes — Core, Glutes

Flexibility	Flexibility
★☆☆	★☆☆

🕐 Keep at it for 5–10 minutes

ON THE EDGE

Your lover hooks their thighs over yours
and dangles their head off the bed.
You enter deeply and give them a
helping hand.

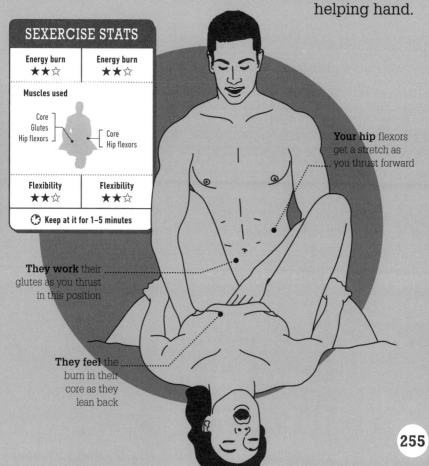

SEXERCISE STATS

Energy burn ★★☆	Energy burn ★★☆

Muscles used

Core
Glutes
Hip flexors

Core
Hip flexors

Flexibility ★★☆	Flexibility ★★☆

🕐 Keep at it for 1–5 minutes

Your hip flexors get a stretch as you thrust forward

They work their glutes as you thrust in this position

They feel the burn in their core as they lean back

255

HALF-PRESSED PASSION

Walk your feet up your lover's body, then beckon them in. Stretching your leg out creates new sensations for you both.

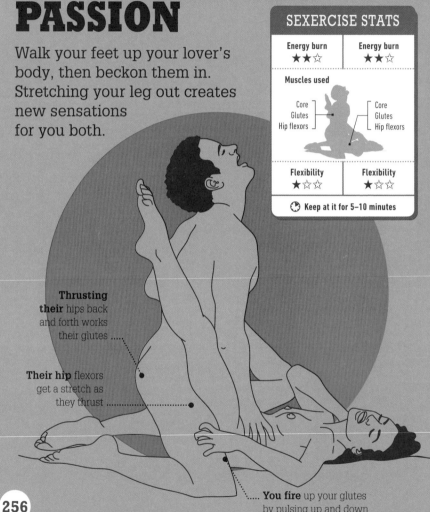

SEXERCISE STATS

Energy burn	Energy burn
★★☆	★★☆

Muscles used

Core Glutes Hip flexors	Core Glutes Hip flexors

Flexibility	Flexibility
★☆☆	★☆☆

🕐 **Keep at it for 5–10 minutes**

Thrusting their hips back and forth works their glutes

Their hip flexors get a stretch as they thrust

You fire up your glutes by pulsing up and down

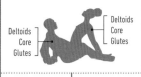
ELEGANT ENCOUNTER

Enjoy the breathtaking feeling of being clasped firmly by your lover. Drawing your feet in behind their buttocks brings you even closer.

You stretch your deltoids as you lean backward

Their core works to keep them stable

The longer you rock back and forth, the more you feel the burn in your glutes

257

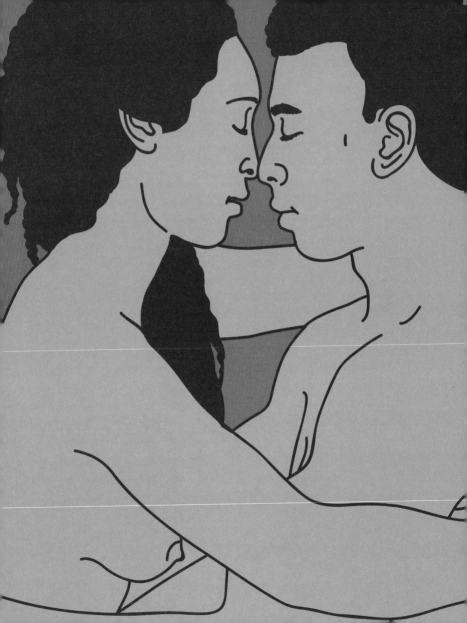

" **IF YOU THEN OBSERVE THE PROPER** *movements* **THEY WILL EXPERIENCE A PLEASURE WHICH WILL SATISFY ALL THEIR** *desires* "

THE PERFUMED GARDEN

DIRTY DANCE

Make this the night of your life. Your lover kneels in front and extends their leg out behind.

You work your glutes as you thrust your hips back and forth

Extending their leg out works their glutes

Supporting their thigh fires up your quads

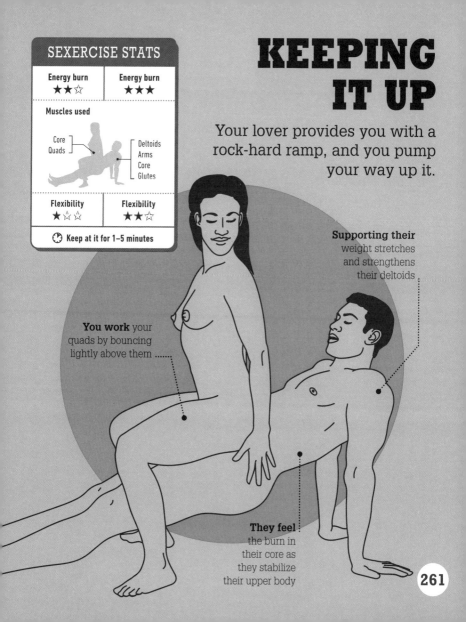

SEXERCISE STATS

| Energy burn | Energy burn |
| ★★☆ | ★★★ |

Muscles used

Core
Quads

Deltoids
Arms
Core
Glutes

| Flexibility | Flexibility |
| ★☆☆ | ★★☆ |

🕐 Keep at it for 1–5 minutes

KEEPING IT UP

Your lover provides you with a rock-hard ramp, and you pump your way up it.

Supporting their weight stretches and strengthens their deltoids

You work your quads by bouncing lightly above them

They feel the burn in their core as they stabilize their upper body

261

TITANIC TINGLES

You might not be face to face, but this pose is still exquisitely intimate. Your lover can breathe gently on your neck or whisper in your ear to make you tingle.

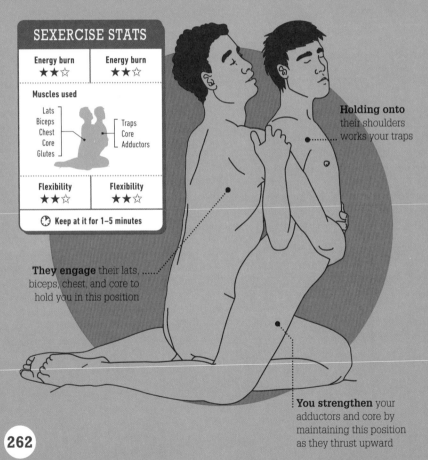

SEXERCISE STATS

Energy burn	Energy burn
★★☆	★★☆

Muscles used

Lats
Biceps
Chest
Core
Glutes

Traps
Core
Adductors

Flexibility	Flexibility
★★☆	★★☆

🕐 **Keep at it for 1–5 minutes**

Holding onto their shoulders works your traps

They engage their lats, biceps, chest, and core to hold you in this position

You strengthen your adductors and core by maintaining this position as they thrust upward

MIRROR, MIRROR

For when you're truly in sync. Match your lover's moves and make each other moan. If you can't balance, use a footstool.

They activate their core to balance on one foot

They work their glutes by thrusting back and forth

They engage their quads to keep themselves stable

SEXERCISE STATS

Energy burn	Energy burn
★★☆	★★☆

Muscles used

Core Glutes Quads Hamstrings		Core Glutes Quads Hamstrings

Flexibility	Flexibility
★☆☆	★☆☆

🕑 Keep at it for 1–5 minutes

IT TAKES TWO

This saucy seated position will bring you both to your knees. Lean back and admire your lover from afar.

Thrusting from the hips in this position tests their core stability ....

.... **The longer** they hold this pose, the more they feel the burn in their arms

They fire up their glutes to push upward

CURLED UP

You sit with your feet between their legs and curl up tight. They thrust gently while you pulse back and forth.

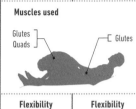

SEXERCISE STATS

Energy burn	Energy burn
★☆☆	★☆☆
Muscles used	
Glutes Quads — ⌐ Glutes	
Flexibility	**Flexibility**
★★☆	★☆☆
🕐 Keep at it for 1–5 minutes	

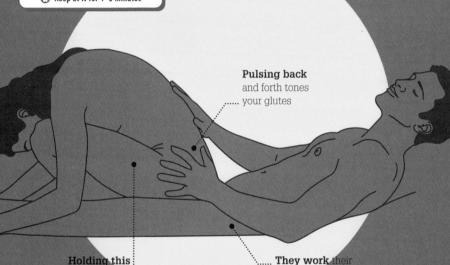

Pulsing back
and forth tones
your glutes

Holding this
compressed position
tests the strength and
mobility of your quads

They work their
glutes by thrusting
up through their hips

LEG TANGLE

Entwine yourselves in each other's limbs and explore exciting new sensations. You don't need to have a foot fetish to enjoy some midsex toe sucking.

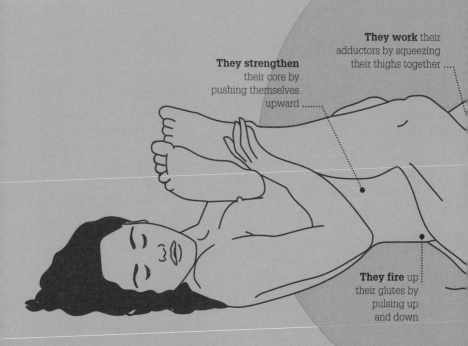

They work their adductors by squeezing their thighs together ....

They strengthen their core by pushing themselves upward ....

They fire up their glutes by pulsing up and down

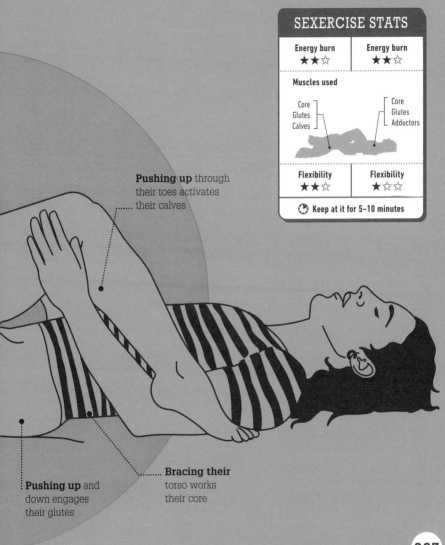

SEXERCISE STATS

Energy burn	Energy burn
★★☆	★★☆
Muscles used	
Core Glutes Calves	Core Glutes Adductors
Flexibility	**Flexibility**
★★☆	★☆☆
🕐 Keep at it for 5–10 minutes	

Pushing up through their toes activates their calves

Bracing their torso works their core

Pushing up and down engages their glutes

267

WIDE OPEN

For when you're feeling flexible and both of you are fired up and ready to explode. Hold your legs apart and both of you get it on.

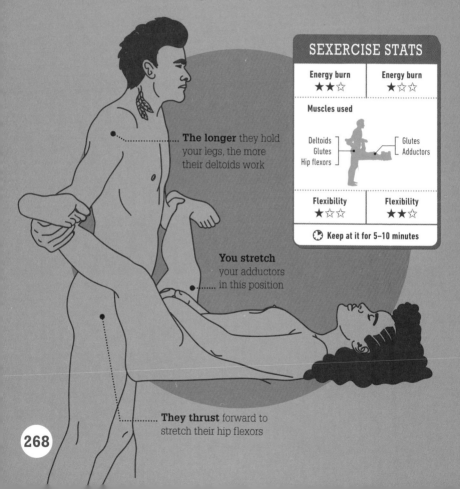

The longer they hold your legs, the more their deltoids work

You stretch your adductors in this position

They thrust forward to stretch their hip flexors

SEXERCISE STATS

Energy burn	Energy burn
★★☆	★☆☆

Muscles used

Deltoids	Glutes
Glutes	Adductors
Hip flexors	

Flexibility	Flexibility
★☆☆	★★☆

🕑 **Keep at it for 5–10 minutes**

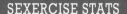

SEXERCISE STATS

Energy burn ★☆☆	Energy burn ★★★
Muscles used	

Deltoid
Glutes
Hip flexors

Core
Lower back
Quads
Hip flexors
Hamstrings

Flexibility ★☆☆	Flexibility ★★☆
⏱ Keep at it for 1–5 minutes	

DANCE RECITAL

Your lover is the prima ballerina in this graceful pose, and you perform the supporting role.

They get a deep stretch in their hip flexors

You fire up your glutes by thrusting back and forth

Balancing on one leg strengthens their quads and hamstrings

269

DOWN ON ONE KNEE

Start by kneeling face to face, then lift one knee and find a flawless fit.

They tense their core to keep themselves stable

Thrusting with their hips in this lunge pose fires up their glutes

They work their quads to maintain this position

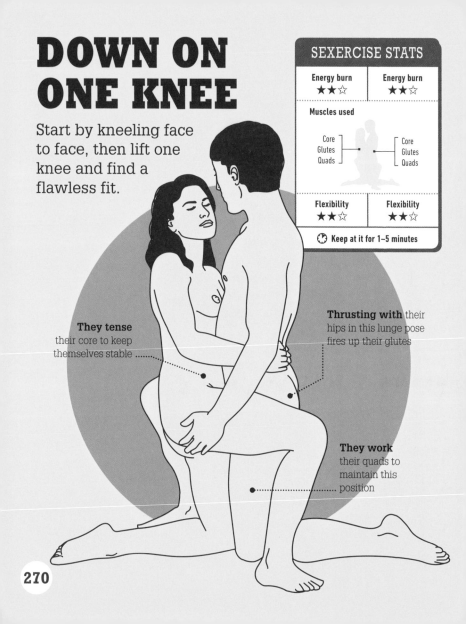

STUNNING HEADSTAND

Your lover rests their head on a pillow and lifts their buttocks high. You get to enjoy the sexy spectacle as you enter.

Thrusting your hips back and forth works your glutes

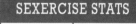

SEXERCISE STATS

Energy burn	Energy burn
★☆☆	★★★

Muscles used

Glutes Quads	Deltoids Core Hamstrings Calves

Flexibility	Flexibility
★☆☆	★★☆

🕐 Keep at it for 1–5 minutes

They strengthen their deep core muscles by stabilizing themselves

They stretch their hamstrings and calves

SIX-▮ACK PLEASU▮E

A cheeky test for those with rock-hard abs: you create a firm slope by pressing your shoulders against a wall, and your lover perches on your lap.

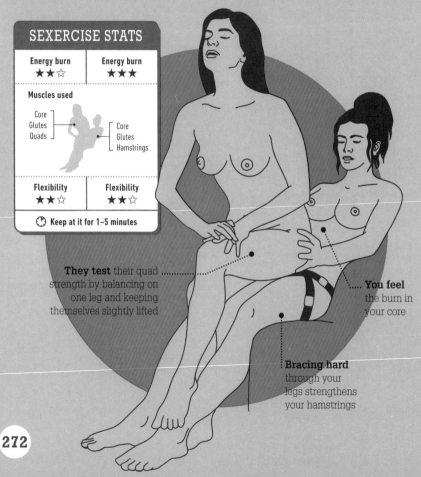

SEXERCISE STATS

Energy burn	Energy burn
★★☆	★★★

Muscles used

Core
Glutes
Quads

Core
Glutes
Hamstrings

Flexibility	Flexibility
★★☆	★★☆

🕐 Keep at it for 1–5 minutes

They test their quad strength by balancing on one leg and keeping themselves slightly lifted

You feel the burn in your core

Bracing hard through your legs strengthens your hamstrings

RODEO ROUNDUP

Kneel over your partner, then they grab your waist and ease you toward them.

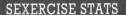
You fire up your core by holding yourself in this position

Holding this pose stretches your hip flexors

Thrusting upward with their hips activates their glutes

TWIST AND TURN

A position with a tricky twist: stay facing away from each other, or your lover can turn around a little at a time until you reunite with a languorous kiss.

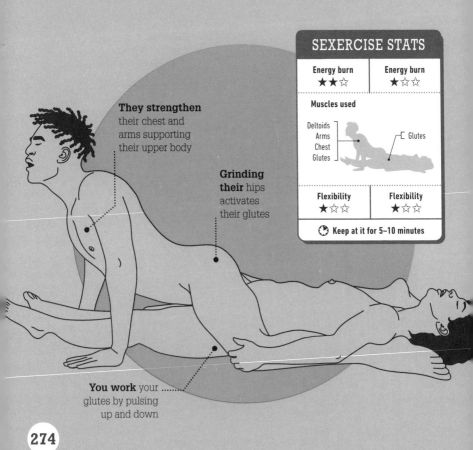

They strengthen their chest and arms supporting their upper body

Grinding their hips activates their glutes

You work your glutes by pulsing up and down

SEXERCISE STATS

Energy burn	Energy burn
★★☆	★☆☆

Muscles used

Deltoids
Arms
Chest
Glutes

Glutes

Flexibility	Flexibility
★☆☆	★☆☆

🕐 **Keep at it for 5–10 minutes**

AT YOUR SERVICE

Your partner traps you between their strong thighs and makes you a servant to their pleasure.

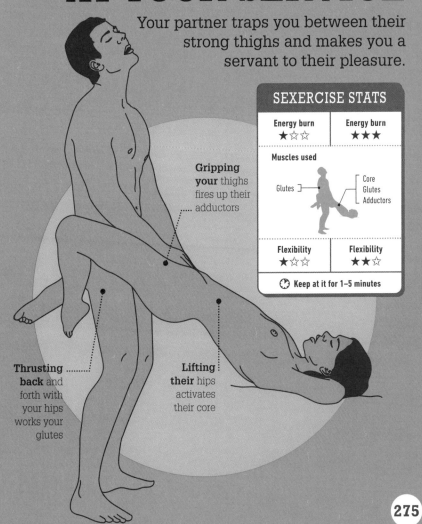

Gripping your thighs fires up their adductors

Thrusting back and forth with your hips works your glutes

Lifting their hips activates their core

SEXERCISE STATS

Energy burn	Energy burn
★☆☆	★★★

Muscles used

Glutes

Core
Glutes
Adductors

Flexibility	Flexibility
★☆☆	★★☆

🕐 Keep at it for 1–5 minutes

275

MUTUAL BENEFITS

You raise your pelvis and invite them to enter. Then you both make the moves, thrusting against each other with abandon.

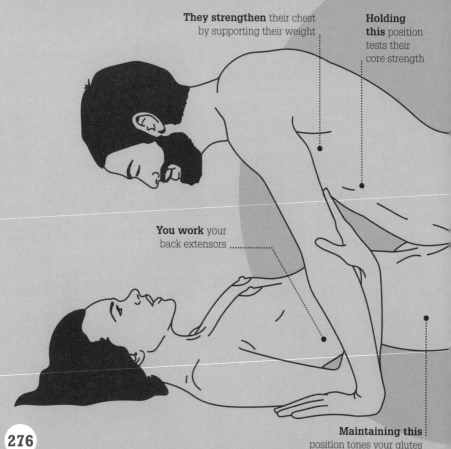

They strengthen their chest by supporting their weight

Holding this position tests their core strength

You work your back extensors

Maintaining this position tones your glutes

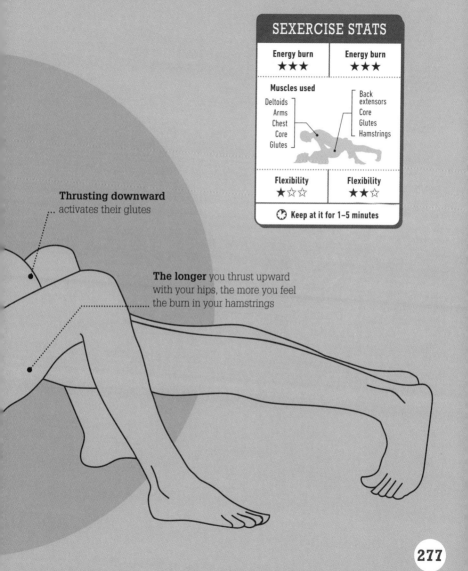

SEXERCISE STATS

Energy burn ★★★	Energy burn ★★★
Muscles used	
Deltoids Arms Chest Core Glutes	Back extensors Core Glutes Hamstrings
Flexibility ★☆☆	Flexibility ★★☆
🕐 Keep at it for 1–5 minutes	

Thrusting downward
... activates their glutes

The longer you thrust upward with your hips, the more you feel the burn in your hamstrings

DIRTY DIP

Clasp your lover's lifted legs and rock back and forth or dip up and down. They can caress your back to intensify the affection.

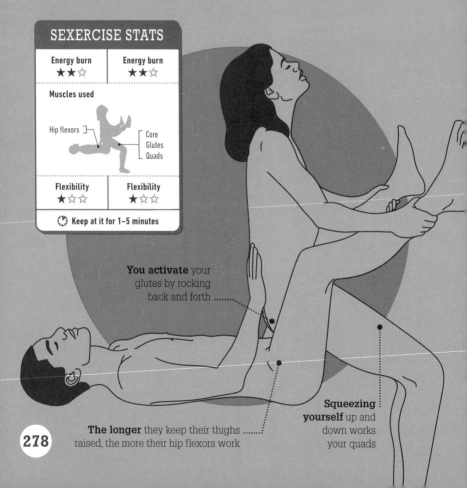

SEXERCISE STATS

Energy burn	Energy burn
★★☆	★★☆

Muscles used

Hip flexors

Core
Glutes
Quads

Flexibility	Flexibility
★☆☆	★☆☆

🕐 Keep at it for 1–5 minutes

You activate your glutes by rocking back and forth

Squeezing yourself up and down works your quads

The longer they keep their thighs raised, the more their hip flexors work

278

STRAIGHT FORWARD

Stretch your legs out long and pull your lover in close. They bounce up to bliss on their tiptoes.

SEXERCISE STATS

Energy burn	Energy burn
★★☆	★★☆

Muscles used

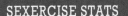

Traps
Core
Quads
Calves

Abdominals
Hip flexors

Flexibility	Flexibllity
★☆☆	★★☆

🕐 Keep at it for 1–5 minutes

Their quads get a workout as they push up and down

The longer you keep your legs up, the more your abdominals work

They work their calves by pushing up on their toes

LOVING ON A PRAYER

Your lover kneels before you and asks if they can enter. You lean back and luxuriate in their display of devotion.

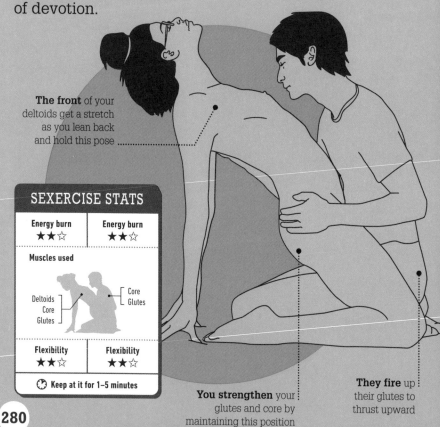

The front of your deltoids get a stretch as you lean back and hold this pose

SEXERCISE STATS

Energy burn	Energy burn
★★☆	★★☆

Muscles used

Deltoids
Core
Glutes

Core
Glutes

Flexibility	Flexibility
★★☆	★★☆

🕐 Keep at it for 1–5 minutes

You strengthen your glutes and core by maintaining this position

They fire up their glutes to thrust upward

HEAD TO TOE

A compact position for cunnilingus aficionados: explore each other's bodies like never before.

SEXERCISE STATS

Energy burn	Energy burn
★★☆	★★☆

Muscles used

Lats
Abdominals
Hamstrings

Flexibility	Flexibility
★☆☆	★★☆

🕐 Keep at it for 1–5 minutes

They engage their lats to hold this pose

Contracting their hamstrings keeps them steady

Maintaining this position works their abdominals

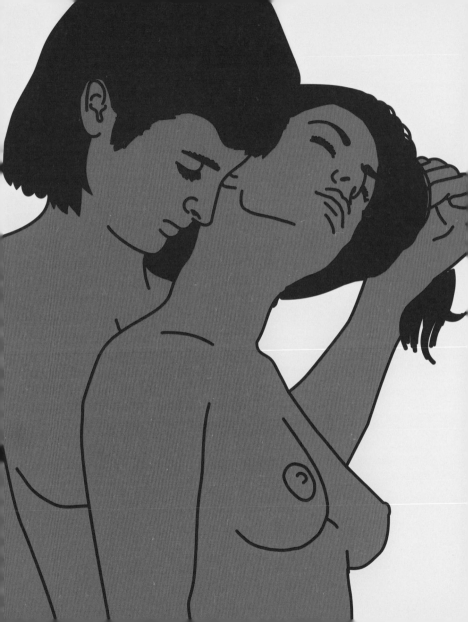

" **TRY DIFFERENT**
WAYS OF
uniting
yourself
TO THEM,
UNTIL YOU FIND THE ONE
WHICH BEST
satisfies
them"

THE PERFUMED GARDEN

HEAD RUSH

They tease you with their tip, then make you gasp as they enter fully. You can dangle your head off the bed for an intense rush.

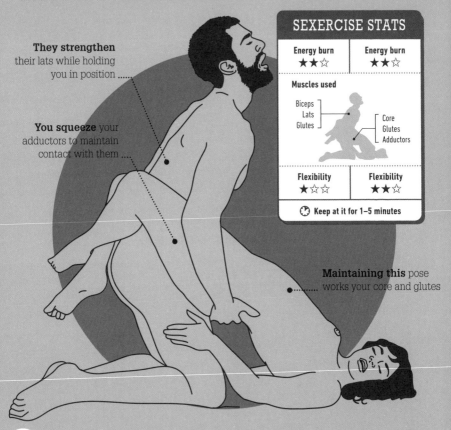

They strengthen their lats while holding you in position ......

You squeeze your adductors to maintain contact with them ...

Maintaining this pose works your core and glutes

SEXERCISE STATS

Energy burn	Energy burn
★★☆	★★☆

Muscles used

Biceps
Lats
Glutes

Core
Glutes
Adductors

Flexibility	Flexibility
★☆☆	★★☆

⏱ Keep at it for 1–5 minutes

ABDOMINATRIX

A scorching-hot position that lets your partner scratch
their love itch however they please. You surrender to
their spellbinding dominance.

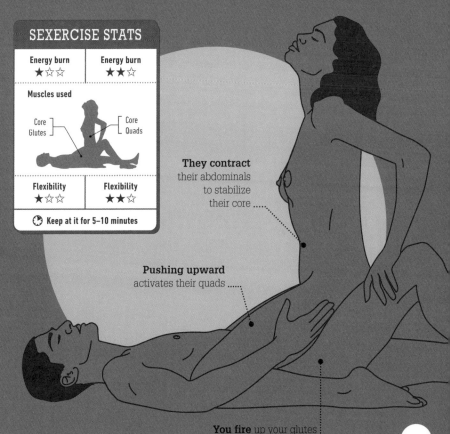

SEXERCISE STATS

Energy burn	Energy burn
★☆☆	★★☆

Muscles used

Core
Glutes

Core
Quads

Flexibility	Flexibility
★☆☆	★★☆

🕐 **Keep at it for 5–10 minutes**

They contract their abdominals to stabilize their core

Pushing upward activates their quads

You fire up your glutes by thrusting upward

HONEY TRAP

Lock your legs around their waist and pull them toward you. They pulse up and down or back and forth to euphoria.

SEXERCISE STATS

Energy burn	Energy burn
★★☆	★★☆

Muscles used

Core
Glutes
Quads

Deltoids
Abdominals
Glutes
Hip flexors
Adductors

Flexibility	Flexibility
★☆☆	★★☆

🕐 **Keep at it for 5–10 minutes**

You work your adductors by holding their waist with your legs

They fire up their glutes by rocking back and forth

The longer you hold this pose, the more your abdominals work

HUMP FOR JOY

Experiment with side-entry sex in this perpendicular position. You cross your ankles elegantly, while they thrust from above.

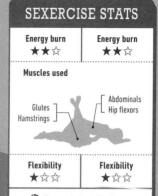

SEXERCISE STATS

Energy burn ★★☆	Energy burn ★★☆
Muscles used	
Glutes Hamstrings — Abdominals Hip flexors	
Flexibility ★☆☆	Flexibility ★☆☆
🕐 Keep at it for 1–5 minutes	

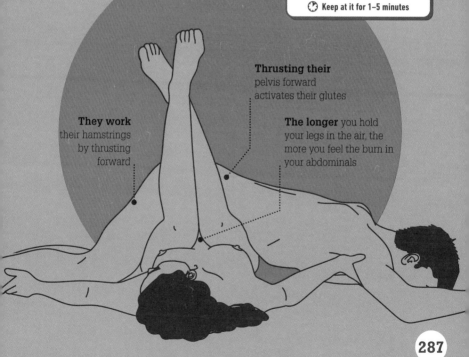

Thrusting their pelvis forward activates their glutes

They work their hamstrings by thrusting forward

The longer you hold your legs in the air, the more you feel the burn in your abdominals

287

BEST FOOT FORWARD

They might be on top, but you're the one in control. You can tantalizingly stroke their chest with your toes or keep them at an enticing distance.

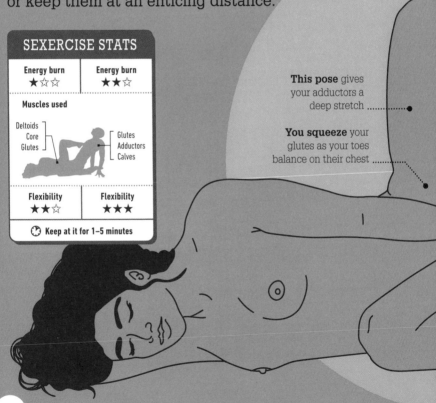

SEXERCISE STATS

Energy burn	Energy burn
★☆☆	★★☆

Muscles used

Deltoids
Core
Glutes

Glutes
Adductors
Calves

Flexibility	Flexibility
★★☆	★★★

🕐 Keep at it for 1–5 minutes

This pose gives your adductors a deep stretch

You squeeze your glutes as your toes balance on their chest

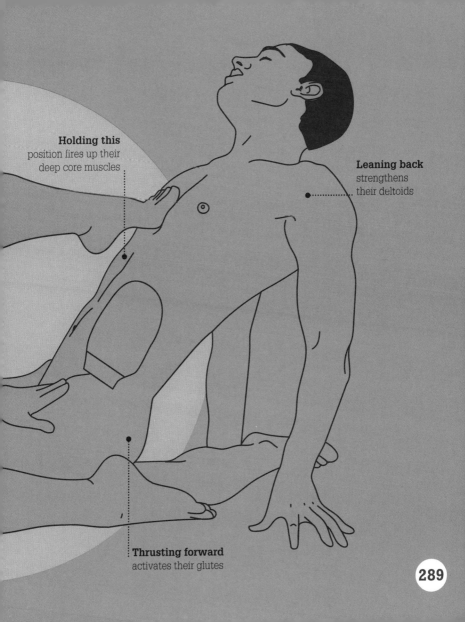

Holding this
position fires up their
deep core muscles

Leaning back
strengthens
their deltoids

Thrusting forward
activates their glutes

289

EASY TIGER

You unleash your inner sex kitten, while they penetrate you at an unusual angle, stimulating unexpected pleasure.

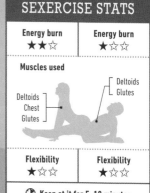
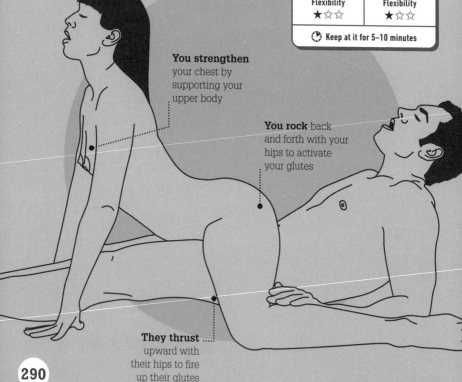

You strengthen your chest by supporting your upper body

You rock back and forth with your hips to activate your glutes

They thrust upward with their hips to fire up their glutes

BUMP IN THE NIGHT

Lifting your buttocks with a pillow lets your lover thrust freely. They can lean in and kiss your neck to up the intimacy.

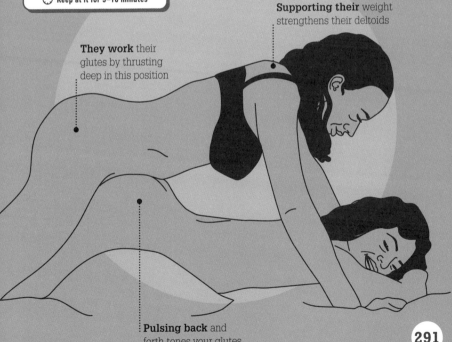

Supporting their weight strengthens their deltoids

They work their glutes by thrusting deep in this position

Pulsing back and forth tones your glutes

POINTED PASSION

Form a solid slope with your body and point your toes perfectly. Your partner slides on and humps their way to heaven.

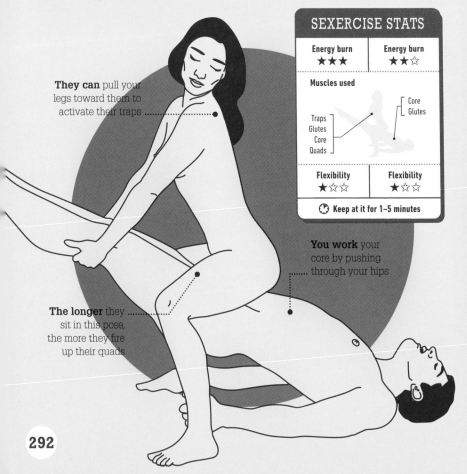

They can pull your legs toward them to activate their traps

The longer they sit in this pose, the more they fire up their quads

You work your core by pushing through your hips

SEXERCISE STATS

Energy burn	Energy burn
★★★	★★☆

Muscles used

Traps
Glutes
Core
Quads

Core
Glutes

Flexibility	Flexibility
★☆☆	★☆☆

⏱ Keep at it for 1–5 minutes

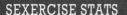

SUPPORTED SUPERHERO

Use your super powers to make your lover soar. If you're both feeling naughty, turn to the dark side.

Energy burn	Energy burn
★★☆	★★☆

Muscles used

Core
Glutes

Deltoid
Glutes
Hip flexors
Adductors

Flexibility	Flexibility
★☆☆	★★☆

🕐 **Keep at it for 1–5 minutes**

They work their core by keeping their torso stable and thrusting through their hips ....

You fire up your .... adductors by gripping their waist with your knees

You strengthen your deltoids as .... you push up against their palms

293

IN BETWEEN

Venture out of the bedroom and into a discreet corridor to put this spicy standing pose to the test.

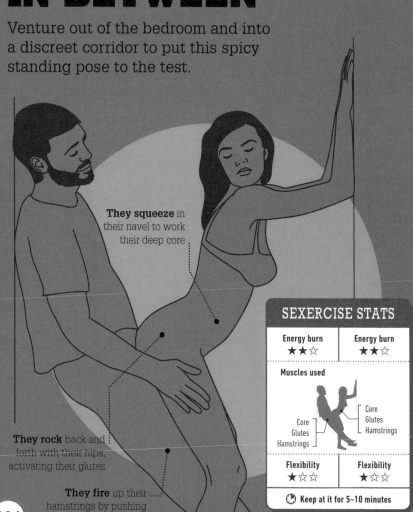

They squeeze in their navel to work their deep core

They rock back and forth with their hips, activating their glutes

They fire up their hamstrings by pushing through their hips

SEXERCISE STATS

Energy burn	Energy burn
★★☆	★★☆

Muscles used

Core
Glutes
Hamstrings

Core
Glutes
Hamstrings

Flexibility	Flexibility
★☆☆	★☆☆

🕐 **Keep at it for 5–10 minutes**

BLIND FUMBLE

Your lover plays the part of a seductive stranger, caressing you from top to bottom. You can clasp their buttocks and pull them in deeper.

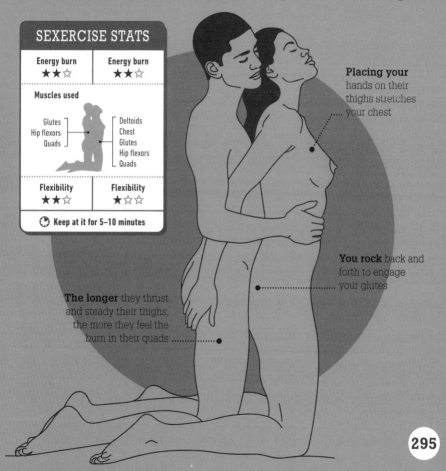

SEXERCISE STATS

Energy burn	Energy burn
★★☆	★★☆

Muscles used

Glutes	Deltoids
Hip flexors	Chest
Quads	Glutes
	Hip flexors
	Quads

Flexibility	Flexibility
★★☆	★☆☆

🕑 Keep at it for 5–10 minutes

Placing your hands on their thighs stretches your chest

You rock back and forth to engage your glutes

The longer they thrust and steady their thighs, the more they feel the burn in their quads

LAZY LOVE

You lie back and let your partner take charge. For extra leisurely loving, you can put your feet on the floor.

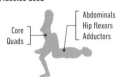

SEXERCISE STATS

Energy burn	Energy burn
★★☆	★★☆

Muscles used

Core
Quads

Abdominals
Hip flexors
Adductors

Flexibility	Flexibility
★☆☆	★☆☆

🕐 Keep at it for 1–5 minutes

You strengthen your adductors by gripping their waist with your calves

Lifting your thighs activates your hip flexors

They work their quads by pushing themselves up and down

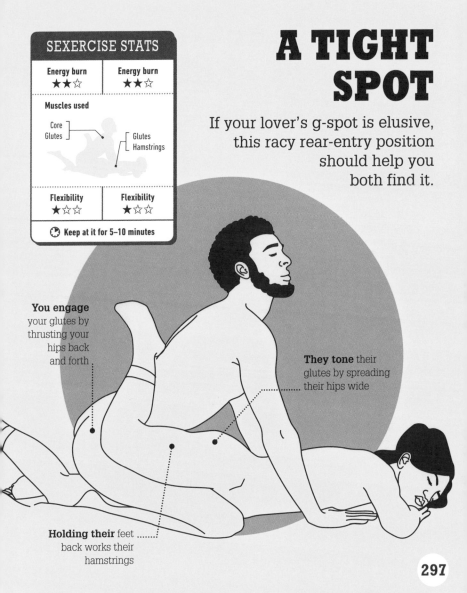

A TIGHT SPOT

If your lover's g-spot is elusive, this racy rear-entry position should help you both find it.

SEXERCISE STATS

Energy burn	Energy burn
★★☆	★★☆

Muscles used

Core
Glutes

Glutes
Hamstrings

Flexibility	Flexibility
★☆☆	★☆☆

🕑 Keep at it for 5–10 minutes

You engage your glutes by thrusting your hips back and forth

They tone their glutes by spreading their hips wide

Holding their feet back works their hamstrings

SLIM HIPPY SEDUCTION

Your lover tucks up tightly and titillates you with the view of their buttocks. You take the bait and slide in.

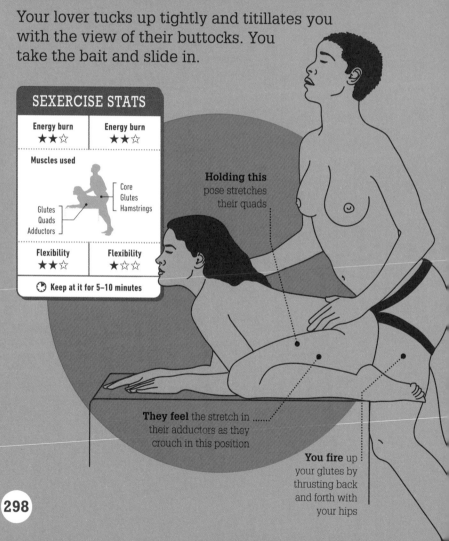

SEXERCISE STATS

Energy burn	Energy burn
★★☆	★★☆

Muscles used

Glutes
Quads
Adductors

Core
Glutes
Hamstrings

Flexibility	Flexibility
★★☆	★☆☆

🕐 Keep at it for 5–10 minutes

Holding this pose stretches their quads

They feel the stretch in their adductors as they crouch in this position

You fire up your glutes by thrusting back and forth with your hips

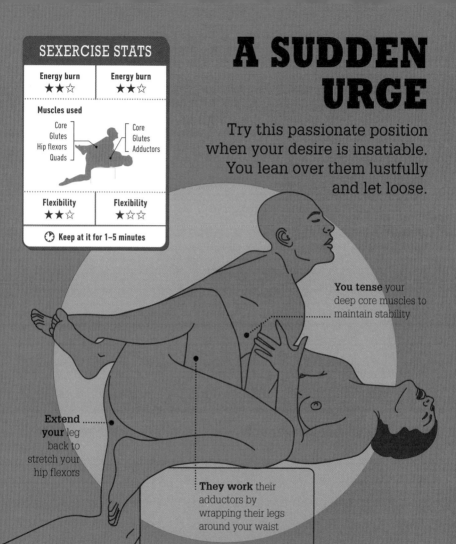

SEXERCISE STATS

Energy burn	Energy burn
★★☆	★★☆

Muscles used

Core
Glutes
Hip flexors
Quads

Core
Glutes
Adductors

Flexibility	Flexibility
★★☆	★☆☆

🕐 Keep at it for 1–5 minutes

A SUDDEN URGE

Try this passionate position when your desire is insatiable. You lean over them lustfully and let loose.

You tense your deep core muscles to maintain stability

Extend your leg back to stretch your hip flexors

They work their adductors by wrapping their legs around your waist

299

ROMANTIC RECLINE

Hug your lover tightly and breathe gently on their neck to send shivers down their spine. Stay in this loveseat or slip into a horizontal position to go at it wildly.

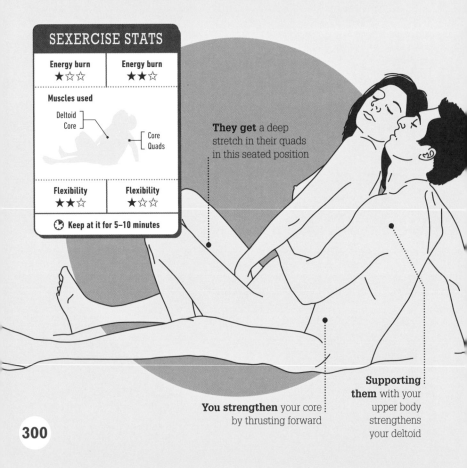

SEXERCISE STATS

Energy burn ★☆☆	**Energy burn** ★★☆

Muscles used

Deltoid
Core

Core
Quads

Flexibility ★★☆	**Flexibility** ★☆☆

🕐 Keep at it for 5–10 minutes

They get a deep stretch in their quads in this seated position

Supporting them with your upper body strengthens your deltoid

You strengthen your core by thrusting forward

BREATHTAKING BALANCE

You bend seductively over an exercise ball, and your lover uses their tongue to knock you off balance.

SEXERCISE STATS

Energy burn	Energy burn
★☆☆	★★☆

Muscles used

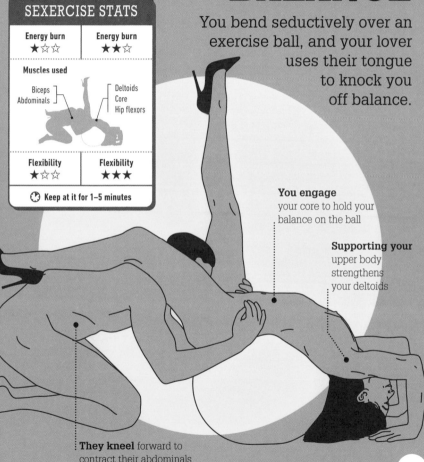

Biceps
Abdominals

Deltoids
Core
Hip flexors

Flexibility	Flexibility
★☆☆	★★★

🕐 Keep at it for 1–5 minutes

You engage your core to hold your balance on the ball

Supporting your upper body strengthens your deltoids

They kneel forward to contract their abdominals

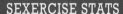
BOTTOM DOLLAR

Perfect for entering from behind. Your lover kneels on a chair, and you penetrate gently.

They can pulse back and forth to fire up their glutes

Maintaining this position works your glutes

You thrust your hips forward to activate your hamstrings

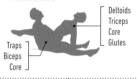
TITILLATING TILT

Begin sitting with your arms around each other. As the sexual chemistry builds, you lean back and lift your legs for a fiery finish.

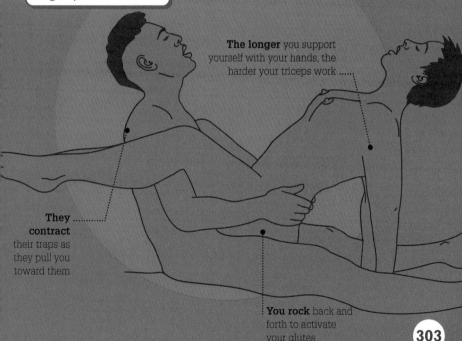

The longer you support yourself with your hands, the harder your triceps work

They contract their traps as they pull you toward them

You rock back and forth to activate your glutes

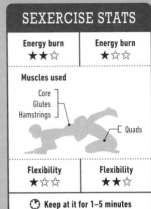

SEXERCISE STATS

Energy burn	Energy burn
★★☆	★☆☆

Muscles used

Core
Glutes
Hamstrings

Quads

Flexibility	Flexibility
★☆☆	★★☆

🕓 Keep at it for 1–5 minutes

PLAYING HARDBALL

Your lover balances impressively over an exercise ball, and you put your mouth to good use.

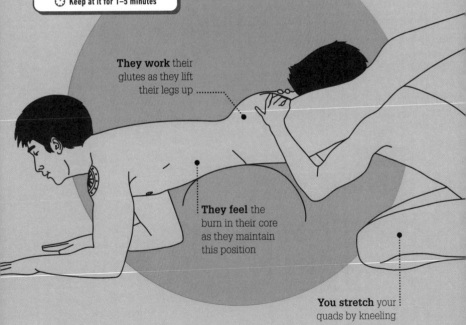

They work their glutes as they lift their legs up

They feel the burn in their core as they maintain this position

You stretch your quads by kneeling

304

HONEYMOONING

Gaze into each other's eyes and lock lips passionately. You pull them close, and they grip you with their leg.

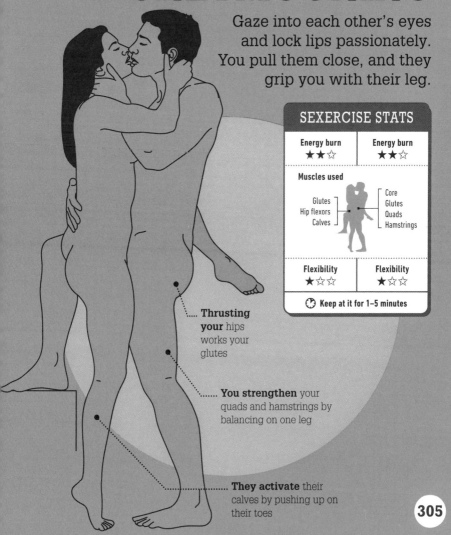

SEXERCISE STATS

Energy burn ★★☆	**Energy burn** ★★☆

Muscles used

Glutes	Core
Hip flexors	Glutes
Calves	Quads
	Hamstrings

Flexibility ★☆☆	**Flexibility** ★☆☆

🕐 Keep at it for 1–5 minutes

Thrusting your hips works your glutes

You strengthen your quads and hamstrings by balancing on one leg

They activate their calves by pushing up on their toes

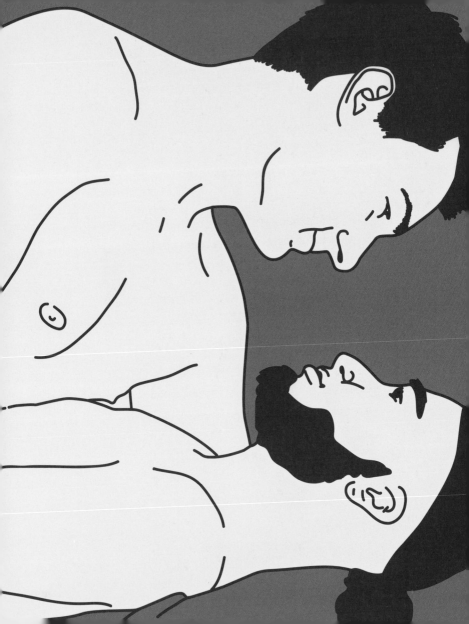

"*The passion* **RESEMBLES A FIRE THAT IS BEING** *lighted*"

ROMEO AND JULIET

Kiss to your heart's content in this position. Pretend it's your last night of passion and make it count.

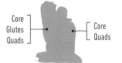

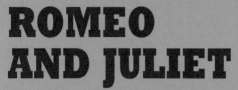

They fire up their glutes by moving in closer

They stretch their quads by kneeling in this pose

Rocking up and down works their quads

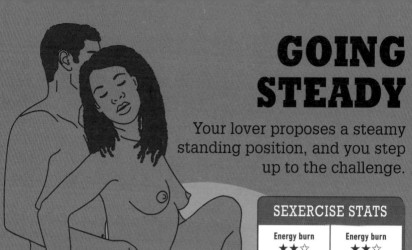

GOING STEADY

Your lover proposes a steamy standing position, and you step up to the challenge.

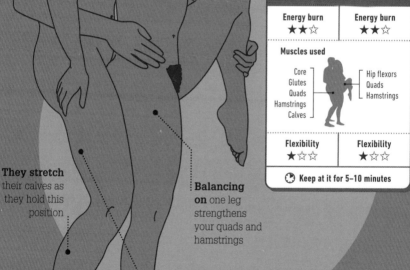

SEXERCISE STATS

Energy burn	Energy burn
★★☆	★★☆

Muscles used

Core		Hip flexors
Glutes		Quads
Quads		Hamstrings
Hamstrings		
Calves		

Flexibility	Flexibility
★☆☆	★☆☆

🕑 Keep at it for 5–10 minutes

They stretch their calves as they hold this position

Balancing on one leg strengthens your quads and hamstrings

Thrusting their hips forward works their hamstrings

309

EROTIC REPOSE

Kneel before your lover and wrap their legs around you. They let you in and press their thighs together for a snug fit.

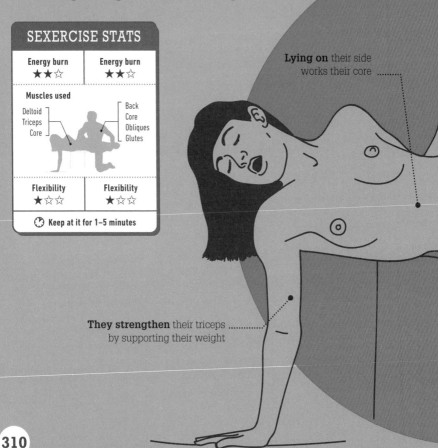

SEXERCISE STATS

Energy burn	Energy burn
★★☆	★★☆

Muscles used

Deltoid
Triceps
Core

Back
Core
Obliques
Glutes

Flexibility	Flexibility
★☆☆	★☆☆

🕐 Keep at it for 1–5 minutes

Lying on their side works their core

They strengthen their triceps by supporting their weight

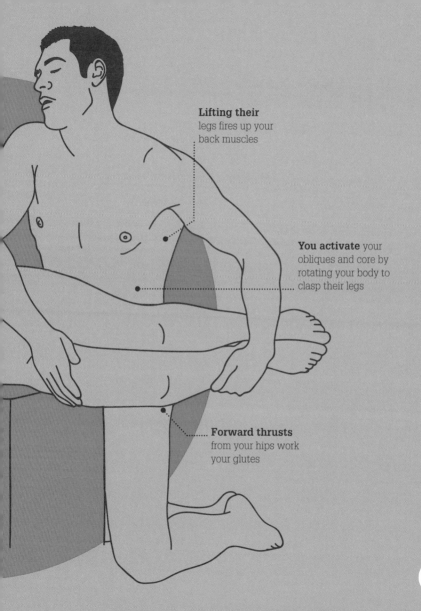

Lifting their legs fires up your back muscles

You activate your obliques and core by rotating your body to clasp their legs

Forward thrusts from your hips work your glutes

LEG EMBRACE

The friction of their thighs on your chest gets you going. They can heat it up for you both by squeezing you inside them.

You activate your hip flexors by thrusting up and forward ....

The longer they keep at it, the more they work their hip flexors

Thrusting upward with your hips strengthens your quads

SEATED 69

If you're feeling creative, try upping your oral game. Hold your lover upside-down to give them dizzying new sensations.

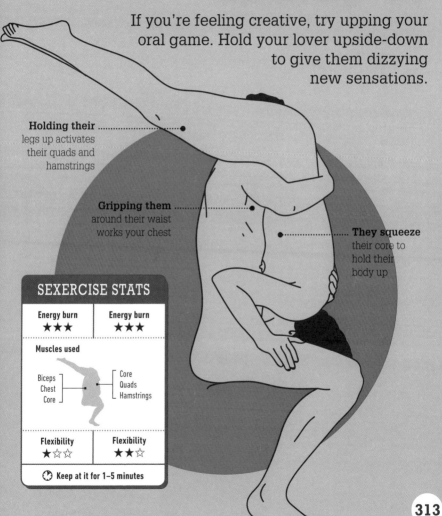

Holding their legs up activates their quads and hamstrings

Gripping them around their waist works your chest

They squeeze their core to hold their body up

SEXERCISE STATS

Energy burn	Energy burn
★★★	★★★

Muscles used

Biceps
Chest
Core

Core
Quads
Hamstrings

Flexibility	Flexibility
★☆☆	★★☆

🕐 Keep at it for 1–5 minutes

THE LEG SPREAD

You both win in this position: the wider your legs can go, the deeper your lover can enter. You put your hands on their chest and rock back and forth.

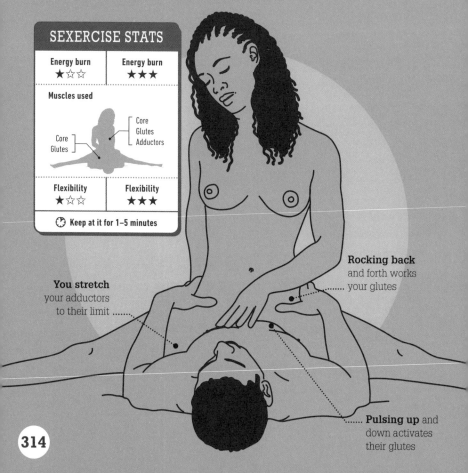

SEXERCISE STATS

Energy burn	Energy burn
★☆☆	★★★

Muscles used

Core
Glutes

Core
Glutes
Adductors

Flexibility	Flexibility
★☆☆	★★★

🕑 Keep at it for 1–5 minutes

You stretch your adductors to their limit ....

Rocking back and forth works .... your glutes

Pulsing up and down activates their glutes

GOING IN DEEP

For achingly deep-reaching sex that is as romantic as it is rampant, you sink in between their thighs and let them pull you in deeper.

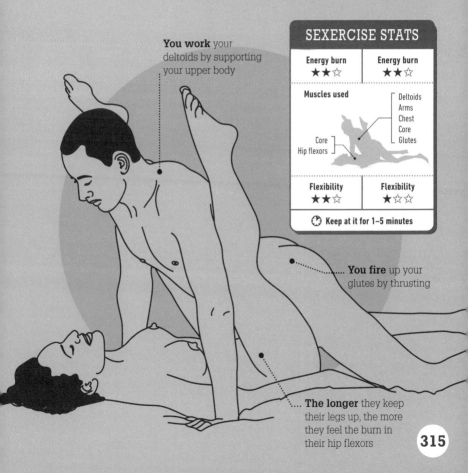

You work your deltoids by supporting your upper body

SEXERCISE STATS

Energy burn	Energy burn
★★☆	★★☆

Muscles used

Deltoids
Arms
Chest
Core
Glutes

Core
Hip flexors

Flexibility	Flexibility
★★☆	★☆☆

🕐 **Keep at it for 1–5 minutes**

You fire up your glutes by thrusting

The longer they keep their legs up, the more they feel the burn in their hip flexors

315

HEATED HOLD

Start with your bodies close, then lean back on your hands and thrust up and down for a fire-cracking finale.

Leaning back
stretches their arms and deltoids

They can
thrust back to strengthen their glutes and core

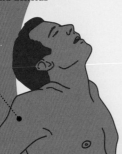

They fire up their glutes to thrust in this pose

316

WEAK AT THE KNEES

Kneel belly to belly and interlock your legs for a divine fit. Turn your attention to your lover's chest: lick, nibble, or bite.

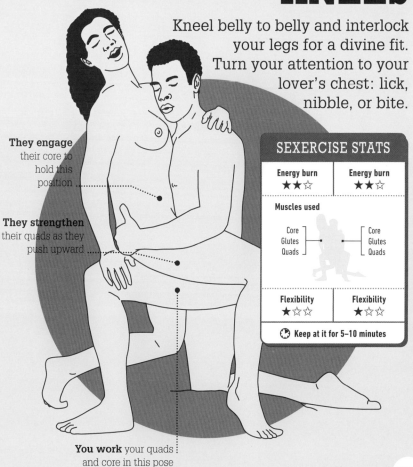

They engage their core to hold this position

They strengthen their quads as they push upward

You work your quads and core in this pose

SEXERCISE STATS

Energy burn ★★☆	Energy burn ★★☆
Muscles used	
Core Glutes Quads	Core Glutes Quads
Flexibility ★☆☆	Flexibility ★☆☆

⏱ **Keep at it for 5–10 minutes**

BEWITCHING BALLERINA

Extend one leg to the side and let your lover lift the other. They can caress your inner calf to make you quiver.

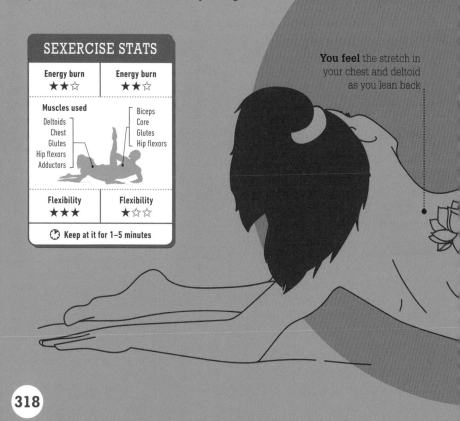

SEXERCISE STATS

Energy burn ★★☆	Energy burn ★★☆
Muscles used Deltoids, Chest, Glutes, Hip flexors, Adductors	Biceps, Core, Glutes, Hip flexors
Flexibility ★★★	Flexibility ★☆☆

🕑 Keep at it for 1–5 minutes

You feel the stretch in your chest and deltoid as you lean back

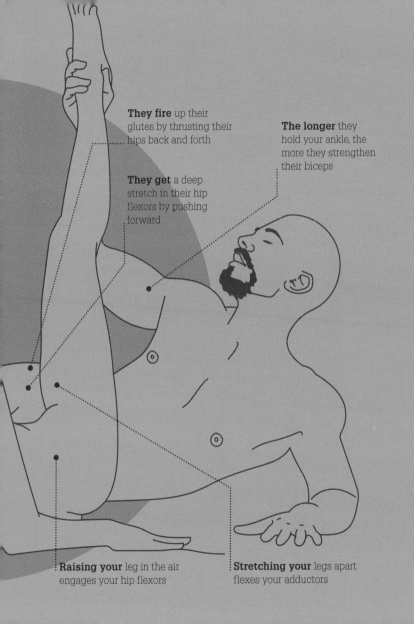

They fire up their glutes by thrusting their hips back and forth

The longer they hold your ankle, the more they strengthen their biceps

They get a deep stretch in their hip flexors by pushing forward

Raising your leg in the air engages your hip flexors

Stretching your legs apart flexes your adductors

319

AIRS AND GRACES

They straddle you seductively, then lean back and slide their hands down your legs. You use your hands to bring them to a powerful peak.

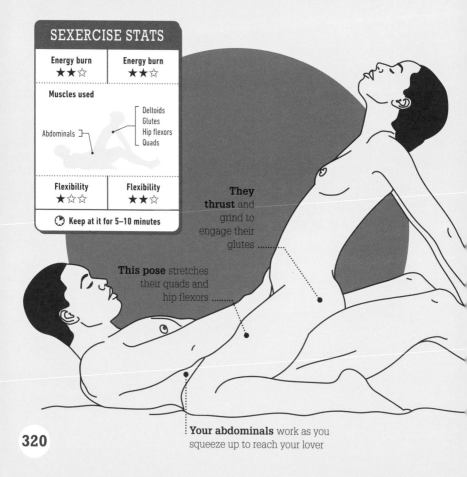

SEXERCISE STATS

Energy burn	Energy burn
★★☆	★★☆

Muscles used

Abdominals

Deltoids
Glutes
Hip flexors
Quads

Flexibility	Flexibility
★☆☆	★★☆

🕑 Keep at it for 5–10 minutes

They thrust and grind to engage their glutes

This pose stretches their quads and hip flexors

Your abdominals work as you squeeze up to reach your lover

HEAT OF THE MOMENT

When your lust is raring to go, grab your lover and pull them in close.

Leaning back works their back extensors

Thrusting with their hips engages their glutes

They pulse back and forth to activate their glutes

SEXERCISE STATS

Energy burn	Energy burn
★★☆	★★☆

Muscles used

Glutes

Back extensors
Core

Flexibility	Flexibility
★☆☆	★☆☆

🕐 Keep at it for 5–10 minutes

FULL TILT

Hold your lover's legs and lean back languorously. They can thrust from below or push your buttocks up and down.

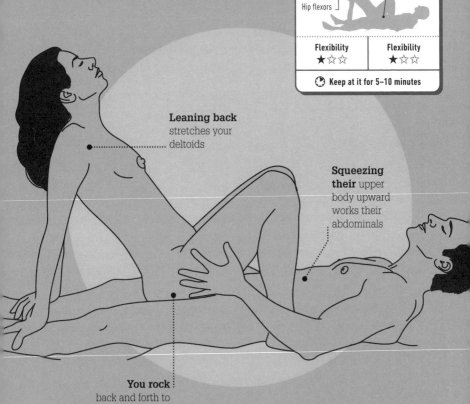

Leaning back stretches your deltoids

Squeezing their upper body upward works their abdominals

You rock back and forth to activate your glutes

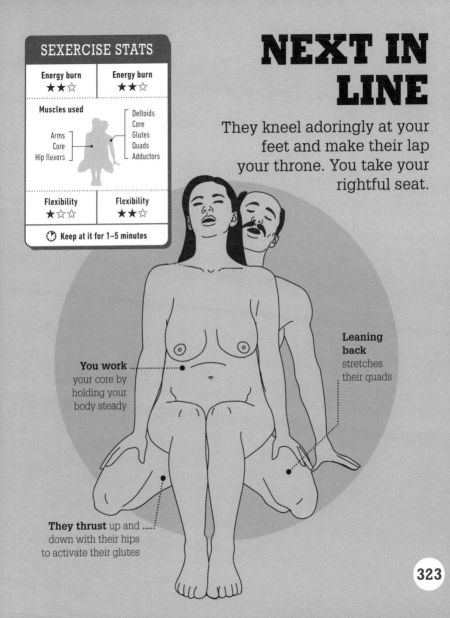

NEXT IN LINE

They kneel adoringly at your feet and make their lap your throne. You take your rightful seat.

SEXERCISE STATS

Energy burn ★★☆	Energy burn ★★☆
Muscles used Arms Core Hip flexors	Deltoids Core Glutes Quads Adductors
Flexibility ★☆☆	Flexibility ★★☆

🕑 Keep at it for 1–5 minutes

Leaning back stretches their quads

You work your core by holding your body steady

They thrust up and down with their hips to activate their glutes

LAID BACK

You start on top, then lie back slowly. Your partner enjoys the titillating view and takes the chance to put their hands to work.

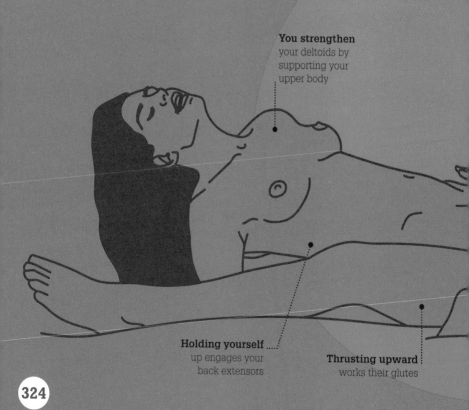

You strengthen your deltoids by supporting your upper body

Holding yourself up engages your back extensors

Thrusting upward works their glutes

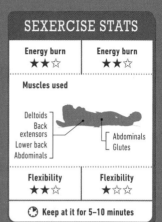

Sliding back and forth activates your glutes

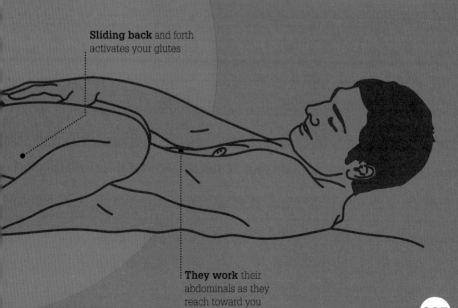

They work their abdominals as they reach toward you

325

BRIDGE OF BEAUTY

Start in a standing position, then lean backward to form a breathtaking bridge.

SEXERCISE STATS

Energy burn	Energy burn
★★☆	★★★

Muscles used

Traps
Biceps
Core
Glutes

Deltoids
Triceps
Core
Glutes

Flexibility	Flexibility
★☆☆	★★★

🕑 **Keep at it for 1–5 minutes**

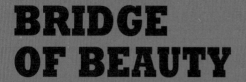

They work their biceps by holding your thighs and waist

You strengthen your triceps by supporting yourself with your hands

Holding this pose tests your core strength to the limit

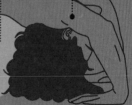

326

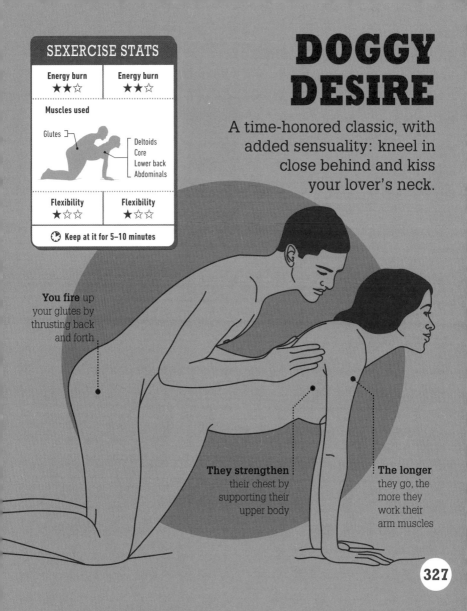

DOGGY DESIRE

A time-honored classic, with added sensuality: kneel in close behind and kiss your lover's neck.

SEXERCISE STATS

Energy burn ★★☆	Energy burn ★★☆

Muscles used

Glutes

Deltoids
Core
Lower back
Abdominals

Flexibility ★☆☆	Flexibility ★☆☆

🕐 Keep at it for 5–10 minutes

You fire up your glutes by thrusting back and forth

They strengthen their chest by supporting their upper body

The longer they go, the more they work their arm muscles

JUNGLE ROAR

Throw yourself at them like a tiger and claw at their chest. They do their best to fight back with their thrusts.

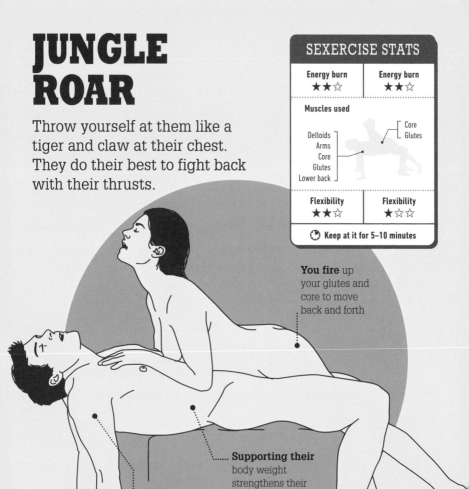

You fire up your glutes and core to move back and forth

Supporting their body weight strengthens their core and lower back

They work their arms and deltoids by holding this position

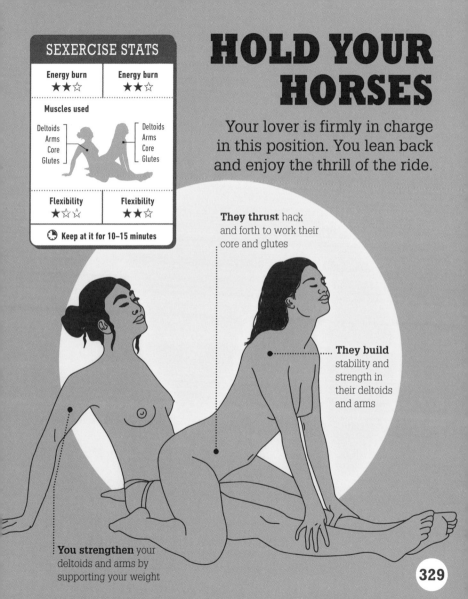

SEXERCISE STATS

Energy burn	Energy burn
★★☆	★★☆

Muscles used

Deltoids
Arms
Core
Glutes

Deltoids
Arms
Core
Glutes

Flexibility	Flexibility
★☆☆	★★☆

🕐 Keep at it for 10–15 minutes

HOLD YOUR HORSES

Your lover is firmly in charge in this position. You lean back and enjoy the thrill of the ride.

They thrust back and forth to work their core and glutes

They build stability and strength in their deltoids and arms

You strengthen your deltoids and arms by supporting your weight

329

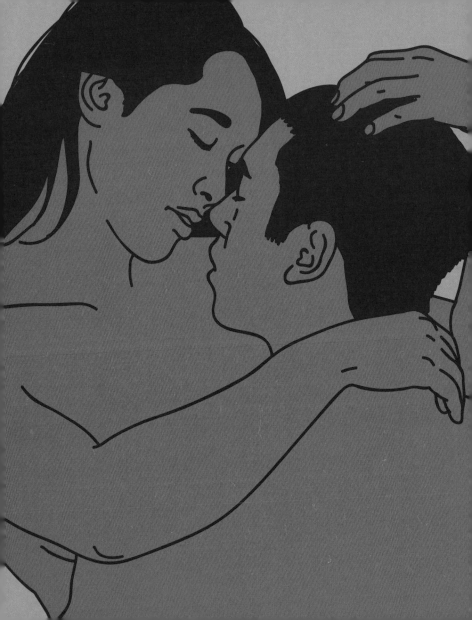

" **WHATEVER THINGS MAY BE DONE** BY ONE OF THE *lovers* TO THE OTHER, **THE SAME** SHOULD BE *returned* "

THE KAMA SUTRA

RAMP IT UP

You are at your lover's mercy, and they take the chance to call the shots. The hot view of their bouncing chest topples you over the edge.

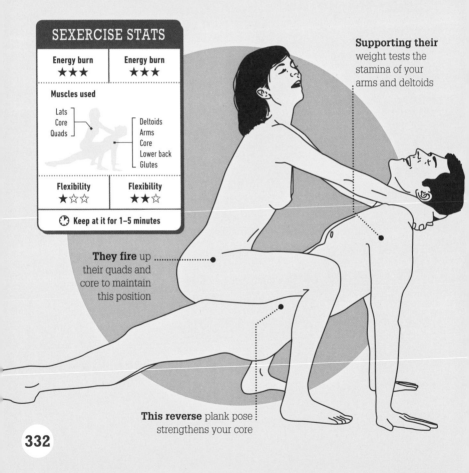

SEXERCISE STATS

Energy burn	Energy burn
★★★	★★★

Muscles used

Lats
Core
Quads

- Deltoids
- Arms
- Core
- Lower back
- Glutes

Flexibility	Flexibility
★☆☆	★★☆

🕐 Keep at it for 1–5 minutes

Supporting their weight tests the stamina of your arms and deltoids

They fire up their quads and core to maintain this position

This reverse plank pose strengthens your core

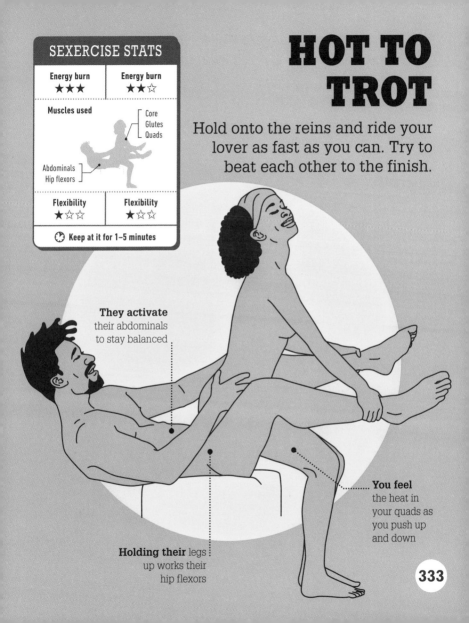

SEXERCISE STATS

Energy burn	Energy burn
★★★	★★☆

Muscles used

Core
Glutes
Quads

Abdominals
Hip flexors

Flexibility	Flexibility
★☆☆	★☆☆

🕐 **Keep at it for 1–5 minutes**

HOT TO TROT

Hold onto the reins and ride your lover as fast as you can. Try to beat each other to the finish.

They activate their abdominals to stay balanced

You feel the heat in your quads as you push up and down

Holding their legs up works their hip flexors

333

WILD WAKE-UP

The perfect way to rouse your partner
from a nap. They open their knees wide,
and you slide in between them.

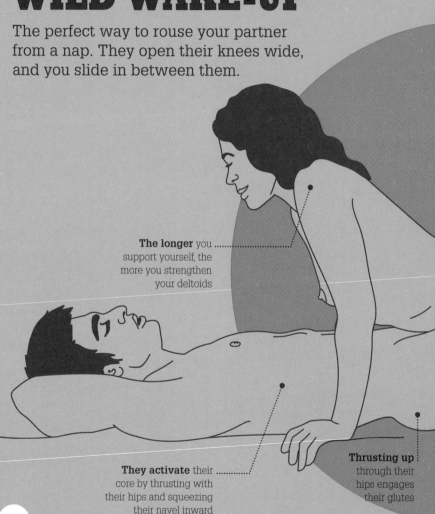

The longer you
support yourself, the
more you strengthen
your deltoids

They activate their
core by thrusting with
their hips and squeezing
their navel inward

Thrusting up
through their
hips engages
their glutes

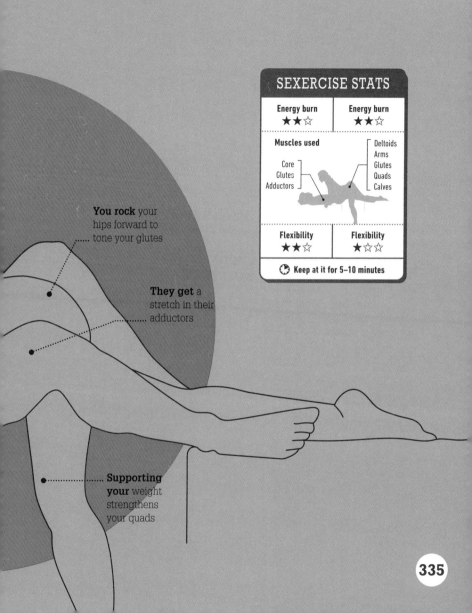

SEXERCISE STATS

Energy burn ★★☆	Energy burn ★★☆
Muscles used	Deltoids Arms Glutes Quads Calves
Core Glutes Adductors	
Flexibility ★★☆	Flexibility ★☆☆

🕐 Keep at it for 5–10 minutes

You rock your hips forward to tone your glutes

They get a stretch in their adductors

Supporting your weight strengthens your quads

335

SULTRY SEDUCTION

You take command in this sexy seated position—they lie back and give you whatever you want.

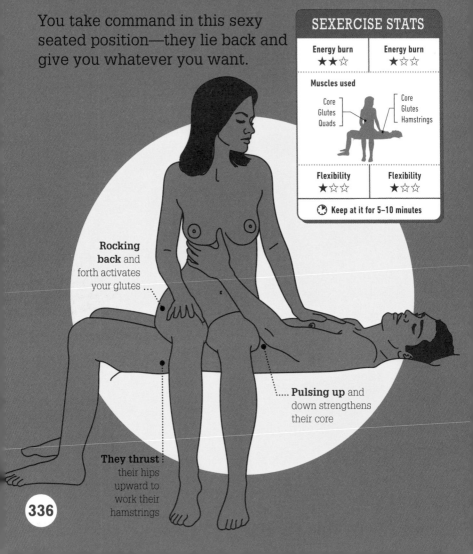

SEXERCISE STATS

Energy burn	Energy burn
★★☆	★☆☆

Muscles used

Core
Glutes
Quads

Core
Glutes
Hamstrings

Flexibility	Flexibility
★☆☆	★☆☆

🕐 Keep at it for 5–10 minutes

Rocking back and forth activates your glutes

Pulsing up and down strengthens their core

They thrust their hips upward to work their hamstrings

HOOKED ON YOU

Get yourselves tangled up in each other: you stretch your leg over theirs and penetrate them from a slight side angle.

SEXERCISE STATS

Energy burn	Energy burn
★☆☆	★★☆

Muscles used	
Glutes Hip flexors Quads	Back extensors Core Glutes Hip flexors Adductors

Flexibility	Flexibility
★☆☆	★★☆

🕐 Keep at it for 5–10 minutes

You get a stretch in your hip flexors

Thrusting with your hips engages your glutes

Pulsing their hips up and down stretches their quads and hip flexors

337

PLAIN SAILING

You are a ship leaning forward to set sail. Your lover thrusts to make the water choppy.

You strengthen your core by contracting your back extensors

They get a stretch in their hip flexors

Rocking back and forth works your adductors and glutes

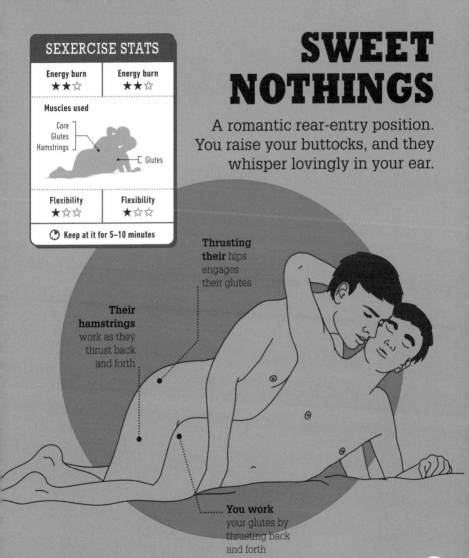

SWEET NOTHINGS

A romantic rear-entry position. You raise your buttocks, and they whisper lovingly in your ear.

SEXERCISE STATS

Energy burn	Energy burn
★★☆	★★☆

Muscles used

Core
Glutes
Hamstrings

Glutes

Flexibility	Flexibility
★☆☆	★☆☆

🕐 Keep it for 5–10 minutes

Thrusting their hips engages their glutes

Their hamstrings work as they thrust back and forth

You work your glutes by thrusting back and forth

INTERTWINED

Get tangled up in each other's bodies and bump and grind freely. Your lover can step up the sensuality by massaging your rear with their heels.

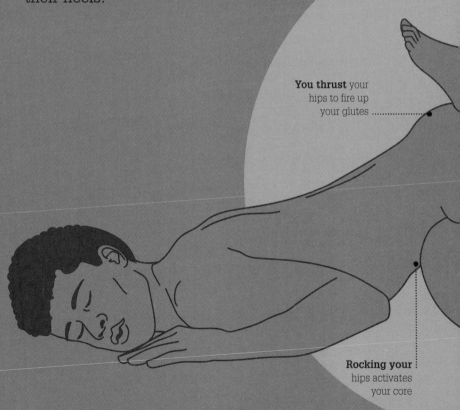

You thrust your hips to fire up your glutes

Rocking your hips activates your core

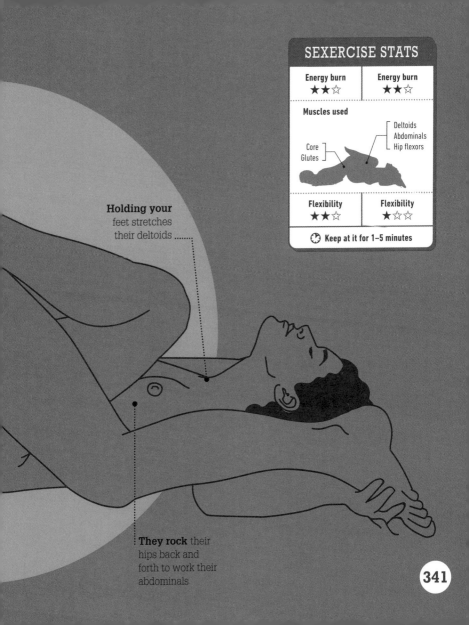

SEXERCISE STATS

Energy burn ★★☆	Energy burn ★★☆
Muscles used	
Core Glutes	Deltoids Abdominals Hip flexors
Flexibility ★★☆	Flexibility ★☆☆
🕐 Keep at it for 1–5 minutes	

Holding your feet stretches their deltoids

They rock their hips back and forth to work their abdominals

341

SEXY SIGHTSEEING

Treat your lover to an enticing view. You can mix short bursts of bouncing with leisurely long strokes to drive them into a frenzy.

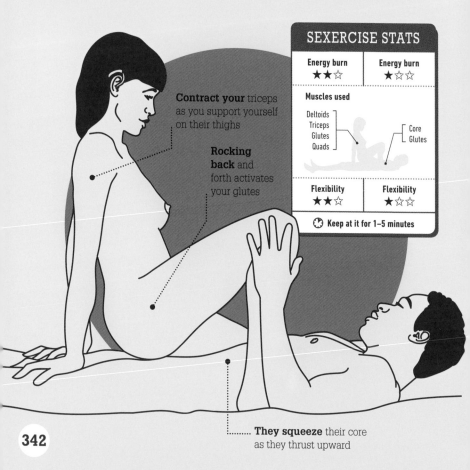

Contract your triceps as you support yourself on their thighs

Rocking back and forth activates your glutes

SEXERCISE STATS

Energy burn	Energy burn
★★☆	★☆☆

Muscles used

Deltoids
Triceps
Glutes
Quads

Core
Glutes

Flexibility	Flexibility
★★☆	★☆☆

🕐 **Keep at it for 1–5 minutes**

They squeeze their core as they thrust upward

SLIP AND SLIDE

Your partner holds onto a chair and rubs on your thigh until you're both on the edge. Slip inside to unleash fireworks.

You feel the burn in your hamstrings as you push your hips up

You squeeze your core hard to maintain this balancing position

Balancing on one leg strengthens their quads and hamstrings

343

HORSE AND CARRIAGE

When your lover's lust is bucking like a stallion, lift your feet above your head and hold them back.

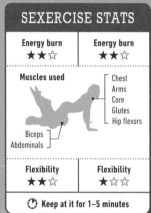

SEXERCISE STATS

Energy burn	Energy burn
★★☆	★★☆

Muscles used	Chest
	Arms
	Core
	Glutes
Biceps	Hip flexors
Abdominals	

Flexibility	Flexibility
★★☆	★☆☆

🕑 Keep at it for 1–5 minutes

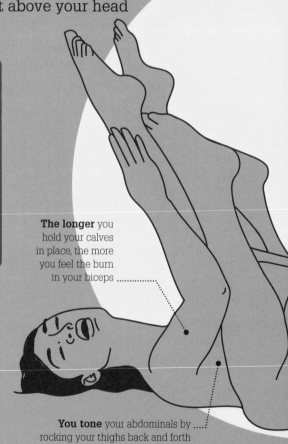

The longer you hold your calves in place, the more you feel the burn in your biceps

You tone your abdominals by rocking your thighs back and forth

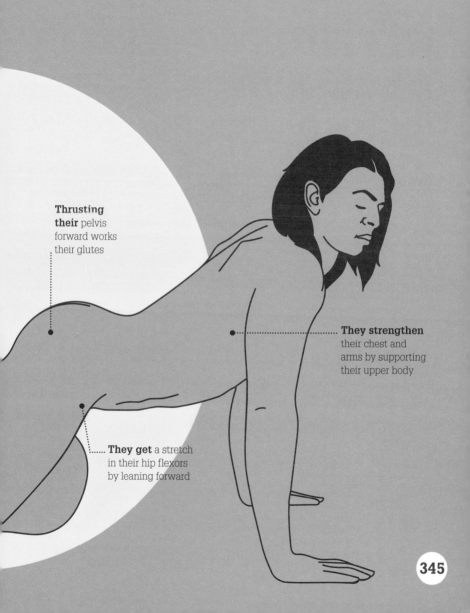

Thrusting their pelvis forward works their glutes

They strengthen their chest and arms by supporting their upper body

They get a stretch in their hip flexors by leaning forward

345

RAVISHING BACK RUB

You give your love a sensual massage, as well as a cheeky something extra between their thighs.

Energy burn	Energy burn
★★☆	★☆☆

Muscles used

Glutes
Hip flexors
Quads

Glutes
Adductors

Flexibility	Flexibility
★★☆	★☆☆

🕑 **Keep at it for 1–5 minutes**

You stretch and strengthen your quads

You fire up your glutes by thrusting your hips forward

Lying in this position stretches their adductors

346

LABOR OF LOVE

This steamy position is worth the effort: you pin your partner with your calves, then they support your waist and lean in.

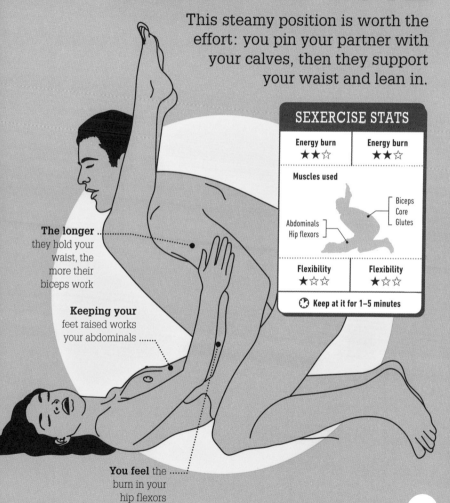

The longer they hold your waist, the more their biceps work

Keeping your feet raised works your abdominals

You feel the burn in your hip flexors

SEXERCISE STATS

Energy burn	Energy burn
★★☆	★★☆

Muscles used

Abdominals
Hip flexors

Biceps
Core
Glutes

Flexibility	Flexibility
★☆☆	★☆☆

🕐 **Keep at it for 1–5 minutes**

SUNNY SIDE UP

Take a different slant on side-entry penetration: your partner lies on their side while you are on your back with your feet in the air.

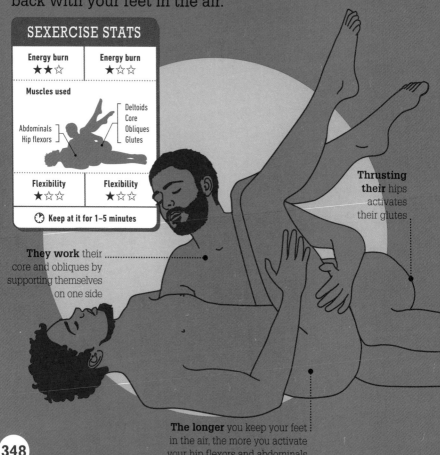

SEXERCISE STATS

Energy burn	Energy burn
★★☆	★☆☆

Muscles used

Abdominals
Hip flexors

Deltoids
Core
Obliques
Glutes

Flexibility	Flexibility
★☆☆	★☆☆

🕐 **Keep at it for 1–5 minutes**

They work their core and obliques by supporting themselves on one side

Thrusting their hips activates their glutes

The longer you keep your feet in the air, the more you activate your hip flexors and abdominals

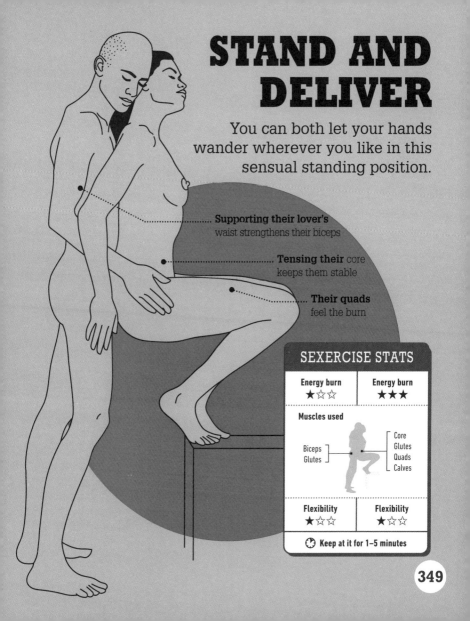

STAND AND DELIVER

You can both let your hands wander wherever you like in this sensual standing position.

Supporting their lover's waist strengthens their biceps

Tensing their core keeps them stable

Their quads feel the burn

SEXERCISE STATS

Energy burn	Energy burn
★☆☆	★★★

Muscles used

Biceps
Glutes

Core
Glutes
Quads
Calves

Flexibility	Flexibility
★☆☆	★☆☆

🕑 **Keep at it for 1–5 minutes**

PERFECT FIT

You wrap your legs around them and control the power of their thrusts. Arching your back and pushing your pelvis up creates a closer fit.

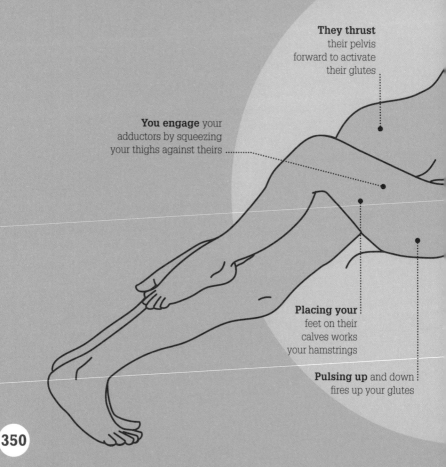

They thrust their pelvis forward to activate their glutes

You engage your adductors by squeezing your thighs against theirs

Placing your feet on their calves works your hamstrings

Pulsing up and down fires up your glutes

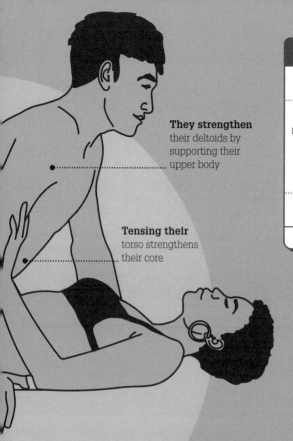

They strengthen their deltoids by supporting their upper body

Tensing their torso strengthens their core

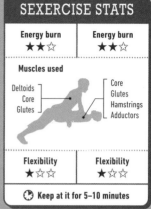

SEXERCISE STATS

Energy burn ★★☆	Energy burn ★★☆
Muscles used	
Deltoids Core Glutes	Core Glutes Hamstrings Adductors
Flexibility ★☆☆	Flexibility ★☆☆
🕐 Keep at it for 5–10 minutes	

BENT DOUBLE

You lean forward in a deep squat, and your partner supports your lower back. Rock to the rhythm of your passion.

You feel the burn in your quads

Rocking back and forth activates your glutes

Holding their upper body in this position strengthens their core

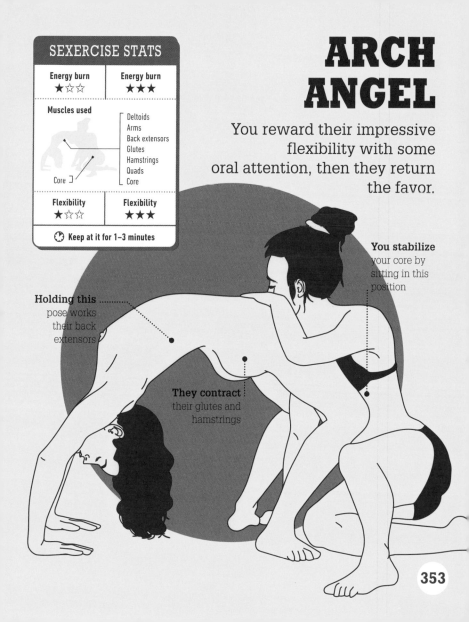

ARCH ANGEL

You reward their impressive flexibility with some oral attention, then they return the favor.

SEXERCISE STATS

Energy burn	Energy burn
★☆☆	★★★

Muscles used	
	Deltoids
	Arms
	Back extensors
	Glutes
	Hamstrings
	Quads
Core	Core

Flexibility	Flexibility
★☆☆	★★★

🕐 Keep at it for 1–3 minutes

Holding this pose works their back extensors

They contract their glutes and hamstrings

You stabilize your core by sitting in this position

353

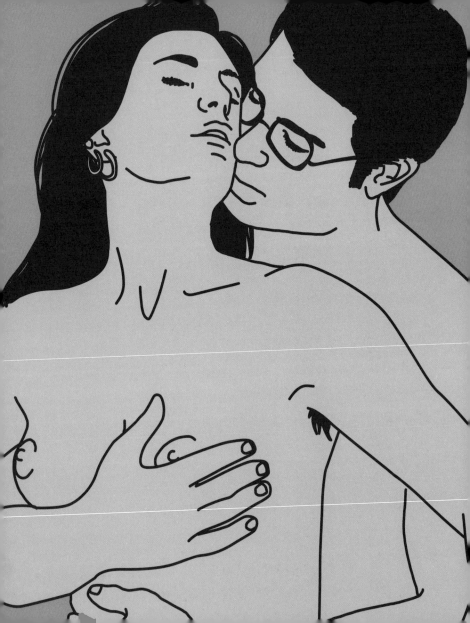

"Prepare them
**FOR ENJOYMENT,
AND NEGLECT NOTHING
TO ATTAIN
THAT END "**

THE PERFUMED GARDEN

STAR-CROSSED LOVERS

You both rock back and forth or thrust up and down to get your hearts pounding in this energetic position.

Their chest and deltoids get a deep stretch in this position

They strengthen their back extensors

SEXERCISE STATS

Energy burn	Energy burn
★★★	★★★

Muscles used

Deltoids
Arms
Chest
Back extensors
Core
Glutes

Deltoids
Arms
Chest
Core

Flexibility	Flexibility
★★☆	★☆☆

🕐 **Keep at it for 1–5 minutes**

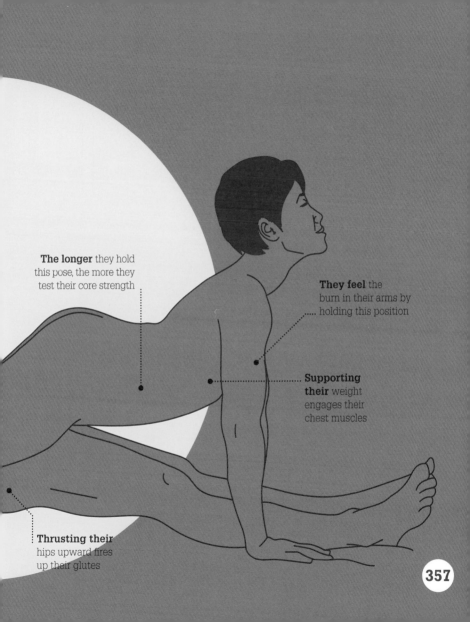

The longer they hold this pose, the more they test their core strength

They feel the burn in their arms by holding this position

Supporting their weight engages their chest muscles

Thrusting their hips upward fires up their glutes

357

CROUCHING TIGER

The ultimate position if you're feeling submissive. You prop yourself up on a pillow, and they enter deftly from behind.

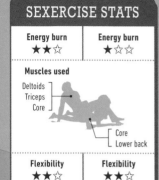

SEXERCISE STATS

Energy burn	Energy burn
★★☆	★☆☆

Muscles used

Deltoids
Triceps
Core

Core
Lower back

Flexibility	Flexibility
★★☆	★★☆

🕐 **Keep at it for 1–5 minutes**

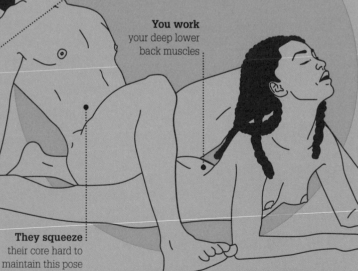

They strengthen their triceps by supporting their weight

You work your deep lower back muscles

They squeeze their core hard to maintain this pose

CHOKE CHAPMEN

A cheeky challenge for the extremely well-endowed: your lover takes a seat on your buttocks, and you aim to enter from below.

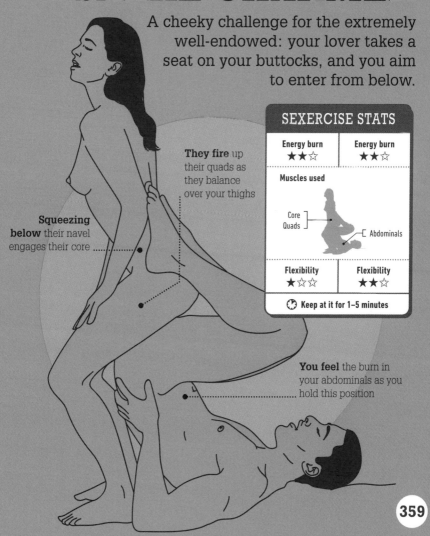

They fire up their quads as they balance over your thighs

Squeezing below their navel engages their core

You feel the burn in your abdominals as you hold this position

SEXERCISE STATS

Energy burn	Energy burn
★★☆	★★☆

Muscles used

Core
Quads
Abdominals

Flexibility	Flexibility
★☆☆	★★☆

🕑 **Keep at it for 1–5 minutes**

A WELCOME SIGHT

Your partner lies back to give you a mischievous view of their whole body. You watch the action from above.

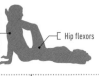
You strengthen your deltoids by supporting your weight

They work their hip flexors by holding their feet on your shoulders

Pulsing your hips back and forth activates your glutes

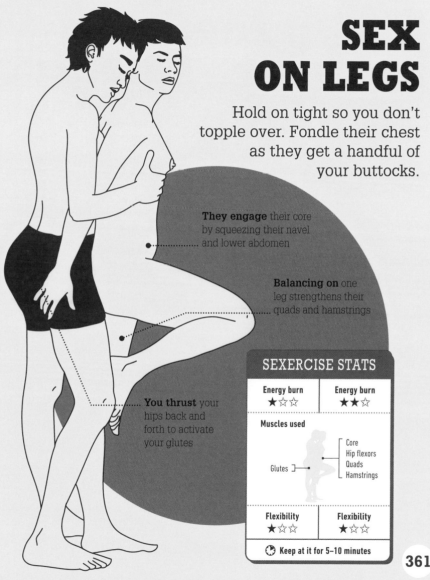

SEX ON LEGS

Hold on tight so you don't topple over. Fondle their chest as they get a handful of your buttocks.

They engage their core by squeezing their navel and lower abdomen

Balancing on one leg strengthens their quads and hamstrings

You thrust your hips back and forth to activate your glutes

SEXERCISE STATS

Energy burn	Energy burn
★☆☆	★★☆

Muscles used

Glutes

Core
Hip flexors
Quads
Hamstrings

Flexibility	Flexibility
★☆☆	★☆☆

🕑 Keep at it for 5–10 minutes

361

ALONG FOR THE RIDE

You clasp them between your legs and take them for a bumpy ride, while they steer you to the finish.

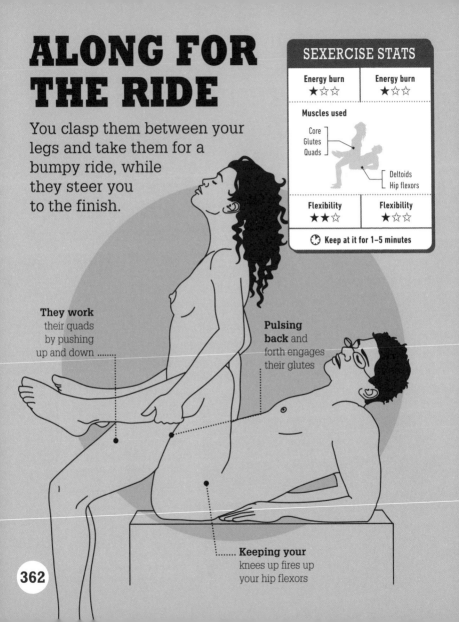

SEXERCISE STATS

Energy burn	Energy burn
★☆☆	★☆☆

Muscles used

Core
Glutes
Quads

Deltoids
Hip flexors

Flexibility	Flexibility
★★☆	★☆☆

🕐 Keep at it for 1–5 minutes

They work their quads by pushing up and down

Pulsing back and forth engages their glutes

Keeping your knees up fires up your hip flexors

CE AMI ATIO

You are in prime position for your lover to investigate as many erogenous zones as they can.

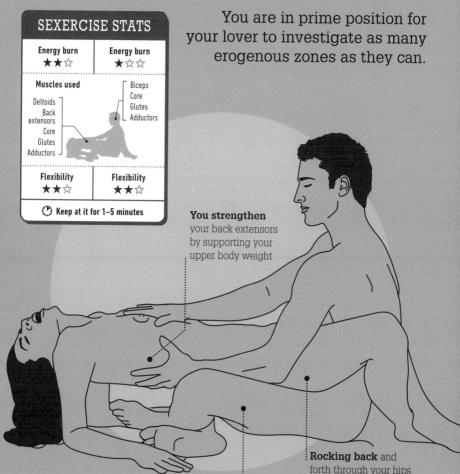

You strengthen your back extensors by supporting your upper body weight

Rocking back and forth through your hips works your glutes

They stretch their adductors by sitting in this position

363

LOVING IN THE AIR

This position is all about you feeling amazing and looking divine. You reward your lover with the loudest moans you can muster.

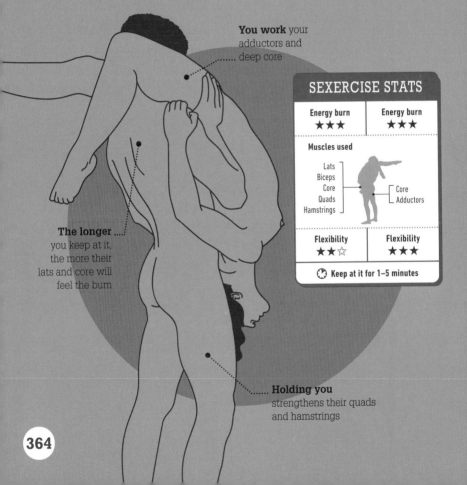

You work your adductors and deep core

The longer you keep at it, the more their lats and core will feel the burn

Holding you strengthens their quads and hamstrings

SEXERCISE STATS

Energy burn ★★★	Energy burn ★★★

Muscles used

Lats
Biceps
Core
Quads
Hamstrings

Core
Adductors

Flexibility ★★☆	Flexibility ★★★

🕑 Keep at it for 1–5 minutes

IGH AND MIG TY

Your partner loves the feeling of being held in your strong arms. Even the minutest movements feel mind-blowing in this erotically taut position.

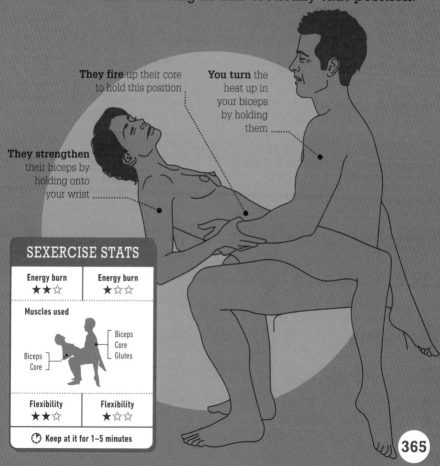

They fire up their core to hold this position

You turn the heat up in your biceps by holding them

They strengthen their biceps by holding onto your wrist

SEXERCISE STATS

Energy burn	Energy burn
★★☆	★☆☆

Muscles used

Biceps
Core
Glutes

Biceps
Core

Flexibility	Flexibility
★★☆	★☆☆

🕐 Keep at it for 1–5 minutes

365

UP CLOSE AND PERSONAL

In this smolderingly sensual position, you each have one leg lifted and one on the ground, so your bodies slot together smoothly.

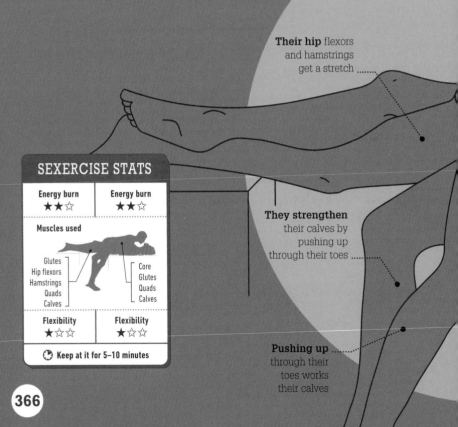

Their hip flexors and hamstrings get a stretch

They strengthen their calves by pushing up through their toes

Pushing up through their toes works their calves

SEXERCISE STATS

Energy burn	Energy burn
★★☆	★★☆

Muscles used

Glutes
Hip flexrors
Hamstrings
Quads
Calves

Core
Glutes
Quads
Calves

Flexibility	Flexibility
★☆☆	★☆☆

🕐 Keep at it for 5–10 minutes

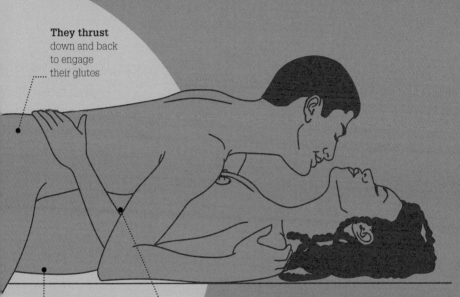

They thrust down and back to engage their glutes

Pulsing their hips up and down activates their glutes

They squeeze their navel and strengthen their core

367

CORRIDOR CUDDLE

You create a strong seat between two walls, then pull your lover in close. They can turn the heat up by lifting their feet off the floor.

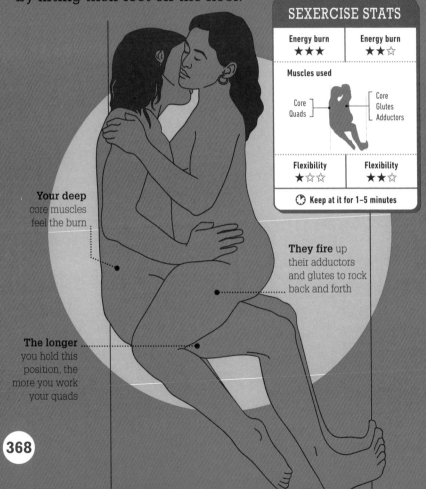

SEXERCISE STATS

Energy burn	Energy burn
★★★	★★☆

Muscles used

Core
Quads

Core
Glutes
Adductors

Flexibility	Flexibility
★☆☆	★★☆

🕐 Keep at it for 1–5 minutes

Your deep core muscles feel the burn

They fire up their adductors and glutes to rock back and forth

The longer you hold this position, the more you work your quads

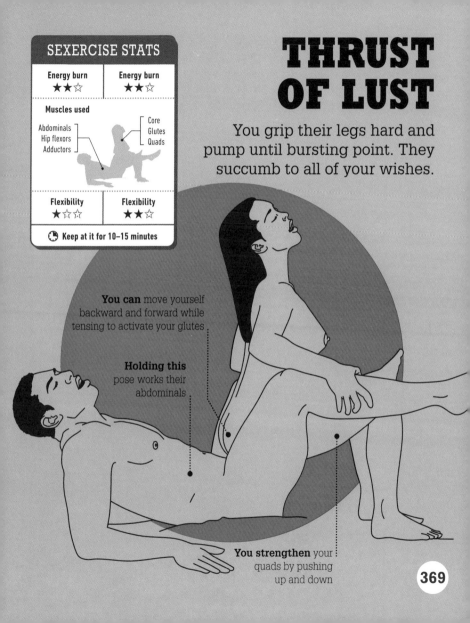

SEXERCISE STATS

Energy burn	Energy burn
★★☆	★★☆

Muscles used

Abdominals
Hip flexors
Adductors

Core
Glutes
Quads

Flexibility	Flexibility
★☆☆	★★☆

🕑 **Keep at it for 10–15 minutes**

THRUST OF LUST

You grip their legs hard and pump until bursting point. They succumb to all of your wishes.

You can move yourself backward and forward while tensing to activate your glutes

Holding this pose works their abdominals

You strengthen your quads by pushing up and down

369

FLEX AND FONDLE

Add some massage oil to this sensuous position to ramp up the romance. Caressing their chest gives them head-to-toe tingles.

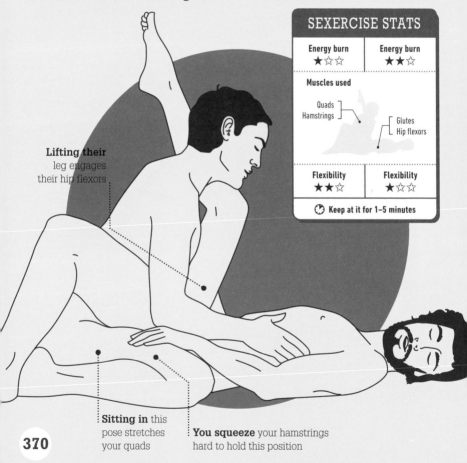

Lifting their leg engages their hip flexors

SEXERCISE STATS

Energy burn ★☆☆	Energy burn ★★☆

Muscles used

Quads
Hamstrings

Glutes
Hip flexors

Flexibility ★★☆	Flexibility ★☆☆

🕐 **Keep at it for 1–5 minutes**

Sitting in this pose stretches your quads

You squeeze your hamstrings hard to hold this position

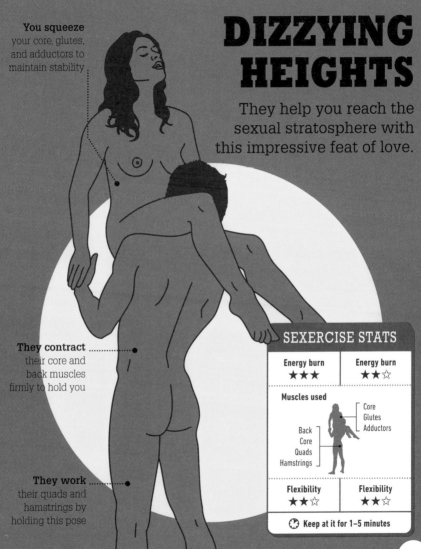

You squeeze your core, glutes, and adductors to maintain stability

DIZZYING HEIGHTS

They help you reach the sexual stratosphere with this impressive feat of love.

They contract their core and back muscles firmly to hold you

They work their quads and hamstrings by holding this pose

SEXERCISE STATS

Energy burn	Energy burn
★★★	★★☆

Muscles used

Core
Glutes
Adductors

Back
Core
Quads
Hamstrings

Flexibility	Flexibility
★★☆	★★☆

🕐 Keep at it for 1–5 minutes

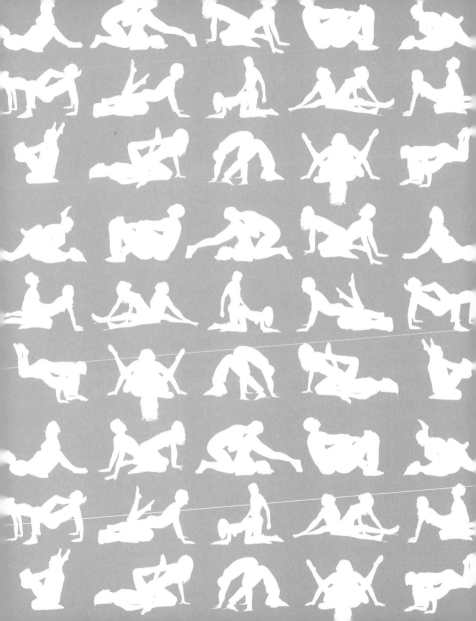

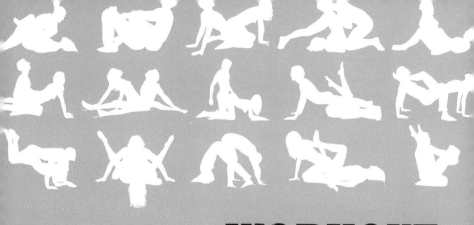

WORKOUT CHOOSERS

Complete a sex session workout by following a sequence of 3 positions, or use the position selectors to choose your next sexercise at random.

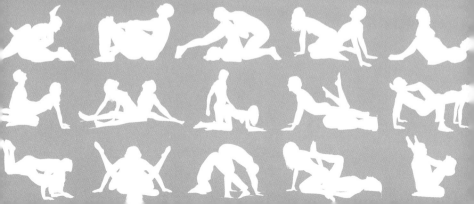

★ SEX SESSIONS ★
ROMANCE

These four workouts are as ravishingly romantic
as they are physically demanding.

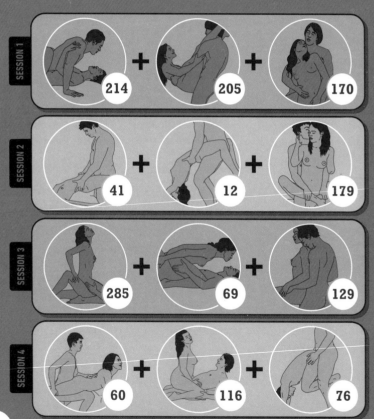

★ SEX SESSIONS ★
NEW SENSATIONS

Pick one of these sexercise routines when you want
to discover out-of-the-ordinary sensations.

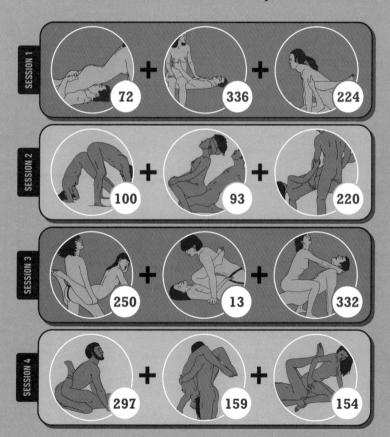

SESSION 1: 72 + 336 + 224

SESSION 2: 100 + 93 + 220

SESSION 3: 250 + 13 + 332

SESSION 4: 297 + 159 + 154

CLOSE ENCOUNTERS

Each of these sexercise sequences gives you the
opportunity for some sensuous skin contact.

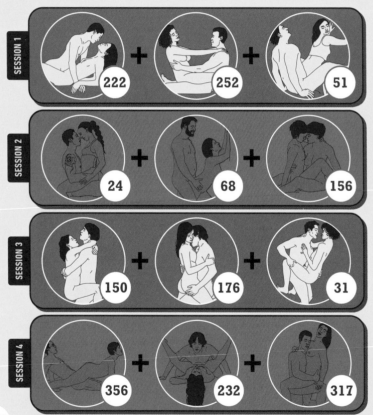

SESSION 1: 222 + 252 + 51

SESSION 2: 24 + 68 + 156

SESSION 3: 150 + 176 + 31

SESSION 4: 356 + 232 + 317

PLAYFUL PASSION

These four workouts are perfect for some frisky
and fun sexperimentation.

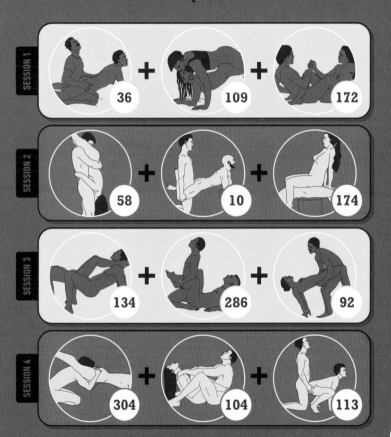

SESSION 1 — 36 + 109 + 172

SESSION 2 — 58 + 10 + 174

SESSION 3 — 134 + 286 + 92

SESSION 4 — 304 + 104 + 113

DOWN AND DIRTY

Choose one of these sexercise sequences
to crank up the kinkiness.

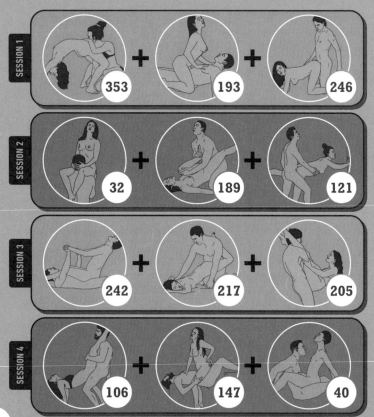

SESSION 1 — 353 + 193 + 246

SESSION 2 — 32 + 189 + 121

SESSION 3 — 242 + 217 + 205

SESSION 4 — 106 + 147 + 40

EXOTIC AND EROTIC

These four workouts will spice up your sex life
and unleash new realms of pleasure.

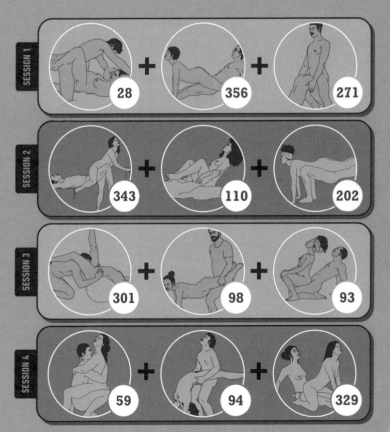

SESSION 1: 28 + 356 + 271

SESSION 2: 343 + 110 + 202

SESSION 3: 301 + 98 + 93

SESSION 4: 59 + 94 + 329

GENTLE

Take potluck with these positions
when you're in the mood for
slow and sensual loving.

129	265	84	360
133	179	155	143
75	180	254	244
362	49	246	161
81	290	26	55

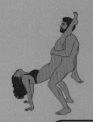
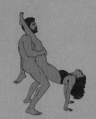

HARD CORE

Pick a pose at random
to get your heart pumping and
your passion soaring.

343	241	83	106
134	332	196	313
237	113	356	276
202	206	250	364
20	92	112	10

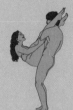
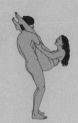

FLEX APPEAL

A lucky dip of steamy stretches:
these positions will bend one or
both of you to the max.

116	205	229	25
288	173	273	137
314	240	233	326
202	318	171	148
208	201	35	134

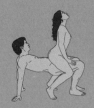

★ POSITION SELECTORS ★

QUICKIES

Forget foreplay: take your pick
of these positions when you
can't wait another moment.

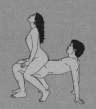

132	144	46	177
365	333	262	60
342	152	57	126
199	238	108	284
96	39	358	82

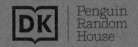

Editor Lucy Sienkowska
Senior US Editor Kayla Dugger
Designer and Illustrator Steven Marsden
Senior Designer Louise Brigenshaw
Jacket Designer Amy Cox
Jackets Coordinator Jasmin Lennie
Senior Production Editor Tony Phipps
Senior Production Controller Luca Bazzoli
Senior Acquisitions Editor Zara Anwari
Managing Editor Ruth O'Rourke
Managing Art Editor Marianne Markham
Art Director Maxine Pedliham
Publishing Director Katie Cowan

This American Edition, 2022
First American Edition, 2018
Published in the United States by DK Publishing
1745 Broadway, 20th Floor, New York, NY 10019

Copyright © 2018, 2022 Dorling Kindersley
Limited
DK, a Division of Penguin Random House LLC
22 23 24 25 26 10 9 8 7 6 5 4 3 2 1
001–332094–Dec/2022

A catalog record for this book
is available from the Library of Congress.
ISBN 978-0-7440-6422-3

All images © Dorling Kindersley Limited
For further information see: www.dkimages.com

Printed and bound in China

www.dk.com
For the curious

MIX
Paper | Supporting
responsible forestry
FSC® C018179

This book was made with Forest Stewardship Council™
certified paper—one small step in DK's commitment to
a sustainable future. For more information go to
www.dk.com/our-green-pledge

ACKNOWLEDGMENTS

For their work on the first edition, the publisher would
like to thank: Paul Persad, fitness consultant.
Dorling Kindersley UK: Alice Horne, Saffron Stocker,
Rehan Abdul, Caro Gates, Toby Mann, Laura Bithell,
Charlotte Johnson, Emily Reid, Robert Dunn, Ché
Creasey, Sonia Charbonnier, Dawn Henderson, Marianne
Markham, Maxine Pedliham, Mary-Clare Jerram.

Paul Persad would like to thank Hannah Schellander.

DISCLAIMER

It is assumed that couples have been tested for sexually transmitted infections. Always practice safe and responsible
sex, and consult a doctor if you have a condition that might preclude strenuous sexual activity. Challenging intercourse
positions might put a strain on your back or other body parts—do not attempt them if you have musculoskeletal
injuries or ailments, and consult your doctor for advice beforehand if you are concerned. Sex in public places should
only be undertaken with due constraints of the law and the sensibilities of others. The author and publisher do not
accept any responsibility for any injury or ailment caused by following any of the suggestions contained in this book.